The Professional Nurse

COPING WITH CHANGE, NOW AND THE FUTURE

Michael Bowman BEd, MEd, PhD, SRN,
NTD(Lond.), RNT, MBIM

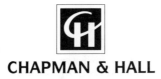

CHAPMAN & HALL

London · Glasgow · Weinheim · New York · Tokyo · Melbourne · Madras

Published by Chapman & Hall, 2–6 Boundary Row, London SE1 8HN, UK

Chapman & Hall, 2–6 Boundary Row, London SE1 8HN, UK

Blackie Academic & Professional, Wester Cleddens Road, Bishopbriggs, Glasgow G64 2NZ, UK

Chapman & Hall GmbH, Pappelallee 3, 69469 Weinheim, Germany

Chapman & Hall USA, One Penn Plaza, 41st Floor, New York NY 10119, USA

Chapman & Hall Japan, ITP-Japan, Kyowa Building, 3F, 2-2-1, Hirakawacho, Chiyoda-ku, Tokyo 102, Japan

Chapman & Hall Australia, Thomas Nelson Australia, 102 Dodds Street, South Melbourne, Victoria 3205, Australia

Chapman & Hall India, R. Seshadri, 32 Second Main Road, CIT East, Madras 600 035, India

Distributed in the USA and Canada by Singular Publishing Group Inc., 4284 41st Street, San Diego, California 92105

First edition 1995

Typeset in 10/12 Times by Cotswold Typesetting Ltd, Gloucester, England
Printed in Great Britain by Hartnolls Ltd, Bodmin, Cornwall

ISBN 0 412 47100 0   1 56593 297 8 (USA)

A catalogue record for this book is available from the British Library

Library of Congress Catalog Card Number: 94-72657

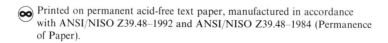 Printed on permanent acid-free text paper, manufactured in accordance with ANSI/NISO Z39.48–1992 and ANSI/NISO Z39.48–1984 (Permanence of Paper).

To my wife Kay and my son Michael for their continued support. To Gregg for his infinite patience. To the many individuals who have influenced and enabled the success of the research on which this book is based. Also, to the numerous professionals who, over the years, guided and influenced my professional development. Finally, to the nursing profession, which I felt privileged to serve.

Contents

Foreword

Michael Bowman's book forms a useful reference source for Health Service staff interested in the role of the professional nurse and the discharge of professional accountability. I am delighted that this work competently deals with nursing's dilemmas about its therapeutic role over a crucial period in its history, especially the effects of major structural change on the profession between the period from the implementation of the Salmon and Mayston Reports up to the present time and Project 2000.

The picture is in Dr Bowman's opinion not a very happy one from the viewpoint of the profession. Some of the changes that have taken place have involved some loss of professional cohesion and were independent of the organizational framework of the National Health Service. Nevertheless, it is disturbing that nurses appear during the period covered to have had a quite inadequate input to the shaping of Health Policy.

There are already signs that the nursing profession has begun to absorb the warnings cited in Dr Bowman's study. However, in the wake of the National Health Service reforms and the implementing of a business culture in the National Health Service. nurses may find the message of this book only too familiar. That does not for one moment mean that the nursing input to corporate strategy and general direction should be defensive or reactionary. British nursing continues to be highly regarded by the general public.

As the political sophistication of the nursing profession increases, I hope that the profession's capacity to think first of those it serves will be dominant in the shaping of the future.

Bill Boland
Senior Quality Officer and Chief Nurse Advisor
North Tyne Health Authority

Acknowledgements

In writing a book of this nature, inevitably the author is obliged to refer to many sources of information to draw upon the expertise of other authors who, over the years, have contributed substantially to the development of the topics discussed. The help and advice afforded me by the many writers and publishers, both in the United Kingdom and abroad, has been unstinted.

I am particularly indebted to Mr W. Boland for reading the manuscript, writing the foreword to the book and offering guidance on the text.

I would also like to thank the nurse managers, ward sisters/charge nurses, staff nurses, doctors and patients of the two district health authorities on which the initial study, which forms the basis of this book, was based, for giving their time and for showing interest in the study from its beginnings. I wish to thank the officers of the nursing statutory and professional bodies, the United Kingdom Central Council for Nursing, Midwifery and Health Visiting, the English National Board for Nursing, Midwifery and Health Visiting and the Royal College of Nursing of the United Kingdom for allowing me considerable time in their busy schedules to discuss key issues of the original study.

I wish to thank Rosemary Morris, Senior Editor, Health Sciences, Chapman & Hall, for commissioning the book and for her generous help and advice throughout the preparation of the manuscript.

I am especially grateful to the following statutory and professional bodies and organizations for their unstinted help in the preparation of the text as well as to the many authors whose work was used in the text, for which permission to publish is much appreciated: the Department of Health, the Controller of Her Majesty's Stationery Office, the publishers of *The Times* newspaper, the publishers of *The Lancet* journal, the Health and Safety Executive, Merseyside, the National Association for Mental Health (MIND), the Royal College of Nursing of the United Kingdom, the Guide Dogs for the Blind Association, the English National Board for Nursing, Midwifery and Health Visiting, the United Kingdom Central Council for Nursing, Midwifery and Health Visiting, the World Health Organization, the International Council for Nurses, the Office of Official Publications of the European Communities, *The Nursing Times*, *Senior Nurse*, *Nursing Standard*, *Nursing Outlook*, *Journal of Nursing Administration*, *Journal of Management Studies*, *Journal of Social Science and Medicine*, *Nursing Research*, *American Journal of Nursing*, *American Sociological Review* and *Administrative Science Quarterly*.

The following is a list of principal sources used in the initial study and preparation of the text, for which permission to publish is much appreciated: D. Warwick, D. Whitmore, H. Mintzberg, M. Quinn Patton and J. Bruner, whose work substantially formed the basis and framework of the methodology for the original study.

Also my grateful thanks to the supervisors of the original study, especially Mr Colin McCabe and Dr Senga Bond, as well as Professor Reginald Revans, Dr Sheila Harrison and Professor George Wieland, Ann Arbor University, Michigan, Dr Adriaan Visser, Director, International Health Foundation, Geneva, for their unstinted advice and support throughout the initial study and to Mrs P. Noons, Nursing Officer with the Nursing Directorate, NHS Management Executive, the many nurse executive directors in NHS trusts who corresponded with me and arranged lengthy interviews regarding current changes, Grahame Walton, Faculty Librarian, Faculty of Health Sciences, University of Northumbria at Newcastle and Ms Sheila Bartlett of CHAT, Royal College of Nursing, for their much valued help.

Preface

This book is based on an exploration of the role of the professional nurse (registered nurse), conducted in two district health authorities. The role of the professional nurse has been much discussed over many decades by different authors in the United Kingdom and abroad. Therefore, why is it necessary once more to undertake further study?

The main aim of the study (Bowman, 1990) was to provide a baseline against which proposals for change could be assessed by analysis and clarification of the role of the nurse. It seemed important to provide an objective understanding of the actual duties, tasks, responsibilities, accountability, authority and autonomy of nurses in order to ensure improved understanding of the reality of their role as perceived by nurses and other professionals and to identify relevant curricula for their education and development.

The methods of data collection used were individual standardized structured interviews together with non-participant observation. The method of analysis was essentially qualitative but some statistical procedures were used in the analysis of the data. The evidence provided by the study is supported by colleagues who are undertaking or have recently completed studies of a similar nature. This indicates that to an extent the findings are not limited to the district health authorities studied but are more broadly based.

The information obtained provides useful data on the nurses' role and the practicality of the Code of Professional Conduct (UKCC, 1984), the continuity, standard and quality of care provided in meeting patients' needs. The data thus obtained enable an appraisal by nurse managers and nurse educationists of the nature of the nurses' role and the related education, training and professional development to meet the needs of that role.

The findings reflect the current debate in the National Health Service on change, resources and standards of care. This book examines and questions whether professional nurses have, over the years, been adequately prepared to enable them to meet, confidently and competently, the challenges brought about by change.

Change

The nurses' role will be affected by much change that has taken place in the National Health Service in recent years, including the new initiatives on Project 2000 (UKCC, 1986, 1987), Framework for Continuing Professional Education and Higher Award, ENB Campus, Communication and Information (ENB, 1992), Nurse Prescribing Formula (NPF) (ENB, 1992), The Scope of Professional Practice (UKCC, 1992), 'Caring for People' (DoH, 1989a) and Self-Governing Hospitals (DoH, 1989b; *NHS and Community Care Act 1990*). Two recent reports by the Audit Commission, namely *The Virtue of Patients* (Audit Commission, 1991) and *Making Time for Patients* (Audit Commission, 1992), identify and amplify many of the findings of the original study (Bowman, 1990). These changes have been heightened by the EEC nursing directives (EEC, 1977, 1989), the Nurses, Midwives and Health Visitors Act 1979, and the Nurses, Midwives and Health Visitors Rules Approval Order 1983. In addition, the influence of reports and legislation to launch the profession into the next century require a clear focus and considerable effort to fit nurses educationally, socially and emotionally for the new demands of their role.

Changing public attitudes, values and aspirations and a better informed public with, as a direct consequence, more demanding patients who are rightfully and properly aware of their rights and needs accentuate the need for a fresh look at the way nurses are prepared to meet these ever increasing demands. The formation of self-governing hospitals, together with the unequivocal statement of patients' rights, as defined in the Patient's Charter, add urgency to securing a sound professional and educational basis for nurses in the effective enactment of their role.

Environment of care: a stressful experience

Nurses work in an environment that was rightfully described by Revans to be 'cradled in anxiety'. The stress, so aptly described in Revans' evergreen *Standards for Morale: Cause and Effect in Hospitals* (Revans, 1964) some three decades ago has been echoed in a catalogue of reports, including *White Collar and Professional Stress* (Marshall, 1980), *Nurse Alert* (RCN, 1984), *Stress* (Hingley *et al.*, 1984), *Stress and the Nurse Manager* (Hingley and Cooper, 1986), and *Motivation, Morale and Mobility: A Profile of Qualified Nurses in the 1990s* (Seccombe and Ball, 1992).

The ever increasing demands of the role of the professional nurse, the level of their responsibility, the nature and extent of their accountability in the context of their perceived limited authority and autonomy to manage their wards and care optimally for their patients, all create much stress and disable nurses, to a greater or lesser extent, in the central execution of their role. This lack of balance in the central, prerequisite elements of their role, highlighted by the study, is compounded by nurses' agreed lack of ongoing professional development.

Nurses continue, with increasing vociferousness, to voice their concerns on the validity, reality and aptness of the trappings of their profession, often including their subordination over the decades to the medical and para-medical professions. Basic to and linked with this chorus of questioning and uncertainty are the aggravating issues of nurses' status, and the lack of true recognition, nationally and by society at large.

Context and philosophy

It is against this uncertain, ambiguous, conflicting and stress provoking background that the text of this book is set. The philosophy underlying the text is based on much extended discussion, formal and informal, with professional nurses, nurse managers, doctors, patients and representative officers of the nursing statutory and professional bodies.

To help the reader engage more closely with and relate more effectively to the findings unfolded in the text, each chapter includes comments on related research and reports as well as specific references.

Even though the title of this book reflects the present and the future role of the professional nurse, the nature of the research study on which the text is based focuses mainly on the present role of the nurse, by investigation and analysis. It uses this baseline, as far as it permits, to justify any prediction on the future role of the nurse, a role which can only be predicted with reservation, when viewed in the context of nursing tradition and the slow pace with which repeated governments and the profession realistically appraise and act on major initiatives, spanning many decades.

Many of the findings of the initial study signalled shortcomings in the way nurses are prepared for their role and the environment in which they work, often limiting the care they are able to give their patients. The picture thus presented is one of pessimism but is entirely based on the perceptions of professional nurses, nurse managers, doctors, officers of the nursing statutory and professional bodies and patients who took part in the study.

Despite this pessimism, it is hoped that initiatives currently gathering momentum, particularly those embodied in the philosophy and framework of Project 2000, reach fruition and launch the nursing profession with confidence and integrity into the next century.

I hope the book affords a measure of satisfaction, pleasure and usefulness to the reader.

Michael P. Bowman

Tables

Appendices

The problem focused | 1

INTRODUCTION

Many reasons prompted the initial study (Bowman, 1990) of the role of the professional nurse (registered nurse), on which this book is substantially based. These included the continuous debate among nurses on the limitations and problems associated with their role.

Nurses perceive the core of the problem to be their workload, with too much to do and too few resources, together with the inordinate pressures of coping with change, organizational and technological; in addition there are the ever increasing demands of informed patients on matters relating to their health, care and progress, with rights enshrined in the Patient's Charter (DHSS, 1991) and 'Statements of Intent' delivered by some health authorities and hospital trusts. Ward sisters and staff nurses commented 'We have the responsibility and accountability to ensure resources, but no authority to enable their acquisition' and 'It is difficult to ensure high standards of care without having control over resources, staffing and materials'. Nurse managers stated that it was their function to initiate and regulate ward resources; nurses were not involved beyond the requisition stage.

Many nurses perceived their education, training and professional development as inadequate and considered that it failed to meet the pressing demands of their job. This failure particularly related to an inadequacy of information and preparation for new developments in relation to their job and the health service as a whole. Their current role demands a full range of skills which include planning, assessing, appraising, budgeting, team building, leadership, monitoring and teaching. To enable nurses to acquire these skills they must be provided with time, resources and opportunity. Ward sisters and staff nurses claim that they 'cannot be freed from work situations because of staffing problems' and that 'lack of money, staff and time prevents staff development'.

Many of these problems and skill inadequacies will be addressed with the progress of Project 2000 (UKCC, 1986). However, there remains at present the majority of nurses who were 'traditionally' trained who need to acquire these skills. This presents its own problems as identified in a UKCC report

(Price Waterhouse, 1987): 'Cost and manpower contraints may prevent Health Authorities achieving this target' (para. 72).

During the study, nurses frequently cited the imbalance between their prescribed duties, responsibility and accountability, questioning the existence of their real authority and autonomy, especially their autonomy to control and make decisions on nursing practice and related matters. For example, many sisters voiced their concern regarding a common practice, over which they had no control, of the inappropriate transfer of patients to their wards due to a general shortage of beds; e.g. patients with acute medical situations were often transferred to surgical wards where often nurses lacked the appropriate skills and knowledge and would have difficulty coping should the patient require emergency treatment. Furthermore, doctors interfered with and sometimes altered established ward care regimes thereby undermining their authority, and they would not accept their advice on the care of patients. The survey of extensive literature and related research on roles in general, and the role of the nurse in particular, enabled the focusing of the study.

CHANGE AND ITS EFFECTS ON NURSES' ROLE

Change in the National Health Service and change in nursing are closely related. The profession of nursing and the framework within which nursing education and most nursing practice takes place, the National Health Service, has been subjected to continuing change, especially during the past two and a half decades. Therefore, it is appropriate as an introduction to the study of the role of the professional nurse to outline the main events during this period that have initiated and/or influenced change in the nursing profession in general and in the role of the nurse in particular.

For example, the 1974 reorganization of the National Health Service (DHSS, 1972) had as its major aim the integration of the major limbs of the Health Service – the hospital, general practitioner and local authority services – to bring about an improved service for patients/clients by ensuring that every aspect of health care be provided locally and with due regard to the health needs of the community as a whole. Regrettably, the reorganization failed in that 'it did not provide the best framework for the delivery of care' (DHSS, 1979, para. 1, p. 1).

Further change took place in 1982 following the publication of the Merrison report (Merrison, 1979), in which the 'Area' tier of management was removed leaving a considerable gap between the district health authority and the regional health authority. The 1982 structural reorganization reflected an earnest and continuing quest for better management, 'to ensure the care and comfort of patients, central to which was the efficient use of resources and the morale of workers' (Merrison, 1979, para. 1.7, p. 2).

The philosophy underlying this reorganization was that intended change should be effected in an evolutionary way, coupled with less central guidance that allowed more local freedom to make precise arrangements. In reality the main effect of the *Health Services Act 1980* was to reduce the many tiers of management that were deemed to be duplicated as well as inhibiting communication and decision making within the NHS. Therefore, as a consequence, it was hoped the new structure would be more receptive to local issues and needs.

Clearly, in the light of much evidence, the changes envisaged and intended by repeated and sometimes extensive reorganization did not fully materialize, as evidenced by the Griffiths Inquiry. However, continued problems plagued the service and, with the publication of the Griffiths report (Griffiths, 1983), further major change was strongly advised to be introduced immediately, allowing little time for debate on a report that continues to have far-reaching effects managerially.

The philosophy of the Griffiths report was thus stated: 'The National Health Service is about delivering services to patients. All that we recommend is the desire to secure the best possible services for the patients' (para. 3, p. 10). The report was critical of National Health Service management and it emphasized the 'lack of a clearly defined management function throughout the organisation and the absence of real continuous evaluation of its performance against criteria such as levels of service, quality of product, productivity, meeting budgets, cost improvement, motivating and rewarding staff'.

The Griffiths report recommendations were ill timed and disturbing, especially the immediacy of its implementation and the emphasis on productivity. In addition, the report brought into question nursing leadership by threatening to deprive nurses of their legitimate right to manage patient services. Administrators were initially hostile to the idea of the appointment of chief executives, understandably seeing their own jobs under threat through appointments from other than the ranks of the administration.

In the wake of the Griffiths report, discontent continues to be voiced by the profession, especially chief officers, mainly due to the fact that they are accountable to general managers/chief executives for the day-to-day perform-ance of their functions. Even though some measure of smouldering discontent continues, the profession, albeit reluctantly by some, have accepted the management framework proposed by the report.

The positive aspects of the report, in addition to making individuals more accountable, could, if effectively implemented, free chief officers of their involvement in the day-to-day working of the service thus enabling them to make more fundamental decisions about health policy.

Change, irrespective of its nature, will affect to a greater or lesser extent the way nurses perform their role. A report (DoH Nursing Division, 1989) indicated the need for change in nurses' role, stating: 'If the role of the nursing profession is first and foremost to respond to human needs, and if in today's world these needs are continually and rapidly changing, then the nursing profession must change with them', and that the goal of nurses must be 'the delivery of health care of the highest standard possible, while taking into account the resources available to them' (paras 1/3, pp. 5/8). These are laudable goals. However, many nurses included in the study experienced difficulty in realizing these goals (a view supported by nurse managers and doctors), stating 'Nurses cannot ensure the privacy, dignity and confidentiality of their patients often because of ward design, e.g. Nightingale type wards and lack of facilities including space between beds, flimsy curtain dividers, enabling conversations between staff and patients to be overheard; lack of toilet and bathroom facilities especially on Longstay and Orthopaedic wards'.

Sisters and staff nurses stated their difficulty in ensuring high standards of care, which they attributed to 'inadequate staffing levels, inordinate administrative workload and dependency on many untrained, unqualified and agency staff'. In fact, when ward sisters ($n = 21$) and staff nurses ($n = 74$) were asked to what extent they could ensure safe standards of practice, 52% and 51%, respectively, stated that they could not do this 'completely'.

How do these acknowledged shortcomings of practice relate to the obligation and accountability as set out in the *Code of Professional Conduct* (UKCC, 1992a)? For example, 'Act always in such a way as to promote and safeguard the well being and interests of patients/clients', and 'Report to an appropriate person or authority, having regard to the physical, psychological and social effects on patients and clients, any circumstances in the environment of care which could jeopardise standards of practice' (paras 1/11).

MULTIPLE ROOTS: HISTORY OF TRADITION

During the initial study, nurses perceived the problems related to their role to have many roots, including the parameters and content of the nurses' role, problems of perception, problems relating to and arising from nursing tradition, social and technological change, the nature of nursing itself, problems of definition and the training, education and development of nurses. Nurses claimed 'basic training is too theoretical. There is no ongoing in-service training relating to the particular problems of ward management and associated new developments and change. Nurses' role is too broad and overloaded'. Staff nurses stated 'The traditional role of the nurse for which many nurses are prepared, is to care for patients. The current role is much more managerially and administratively demanding, but without the necessary support and training'.

The following summary of reports, papers and legislation identified some of the problems and proposed solutions in relation to the preparation of nurses for their role. The Platt Committee (Platt, 1964) was entrusted to consider the whole field of nursing education and training in the light of developments since the work of the Nursing Reconstruction Committee (Horder, 1943). Its recommendations were numerous and far reaching and included vital issues, crucial to the viability and integrity of the profession, relating to the independence of schools of nursing of the hospital service, the pattern of post-registration nursing education, the inadequacy of the existing pattern of nursing education in meeting present-day needs and the difficulty of meeting demands for skilled nursing care within the context of a rapidly developing and increasingly complex service. These recommendations still remain relatively unfulfilled. During the study, 80% of ward sisters and 40% of staff nurses stated their unease regarding 'the regular practice of employing agency nurses, trained and untrained, to bolster inadequate ward staffing levels'. They were concerned about the shortcomings of this policy that 'Far from enabling the care of patients, often because of the lack of knowledge and skills of the nurses thus employed, and their inability (frequently) to meet the specialist needs (skills and knowledge), of the patients for whom they were caring, constituted a potential danger to these patients'.

Research by Revans (1964) into nurse wastage was concerned that communication and information systems in hospitals were poor. He tried to show that 'the interactions between the nurse, the patient and the hospital in which they find themselves are simultaneously both complex and simple', and that 'uncertainty is magnified by communication failure. Unrealistic ideas about one's own role, knowledge, intelligence, status and other features of the self will increase the difficulty of communicating and of being communicated with' (Revans, *Standards for Morale: Cause and Effect in Hospitals*, paras 1/2, p. 91, 1964, by permission of Oxford University Press).

Currently, nurses experience similar communication problems to those found by Revans, in terms of being listened to and/or consulted on matters relating to nursing practice. This point was particularly stressed by newly qualified nurses, many of whom were concerned that their ideas and initiatives went unheeded. The Powell report (Powell, 1966) made it clear that 'if nurses fail to keep up with new knowledge, the lack of understanding which is sure to follow will lead to dissatisfaction, inefficiency and unrest' (para. 8, p. 2). This is fine in theory, but the majority of nurses interviewed complained repeatedly: 'Lack of money, staff and time prevent staff development'.

However, without ongoing professional development it is difficult to see how optimum standards of care as well as the enhancement of the careers of staff can be obtained through sharpness of skills and knowledge. Furthermore, the Code of Professional Conduct imposes on the nurse a responsibility 'to maintain and improve professional knowlege and competence' and, more forcefully, 'acknowledge any limitations of competence and refuse in such cases to accept delegated functions without first having received instruction in regard to those functions and having been assessed as competent' (paras 3/4, p. 2). Nevertheless, 66% of ward sisters ($n = 21$) and 76% of staff nurses ($n = 74$) during interview stated that they could not improve their own professional competence, skills and knowledge.

Problems and their effects continued and many nurses thought that the Salmon Committee (1966) had identified many tasks of which ward sisters could be relieved. These included administrative work and the supervision of domestic staff 'to enable them to give more direct care to the patient' (para 4.2, p. 34). Despite this change nurses continued albeit for other reasons, notably lack of resources and lack of staff, to have limited time to spend with their patients. Many nurses also felt that their authority had been eroded by this very action, because other managers were brought in to supervise tasks and staff which previously were within their remit. The relevance of nurses' authority and the progressively diminishing authority of the professional nurse were discussed by the RCN in three separate documents (RCN, 1981, 1982, 1983) and were confirmed to some extent by the evidence of the sample study.

The Briggs report (Briggs, 1972) reviewed the role of the nurse and midwife and attempted to set the framework for the future training and development of nurses, to ensure the best use of manpower to meet the needs and demands of an integrated health service. It took two years following publication of the report before it was officially acknowledged by the government. In relation to training Briggs recommended: 'There should be improved continuity and co-ordination in classroom and service, with greater involvement of teachers in the service setting' (recommendation 32, p. 214). The report recognized that 'There should be a major drive started as quickly as possible, to produce more nursing and midwifery teachers' (recommendation 35, p. 214). The General Nursing Council was 'unhappy' about the implementation of its major recommendations until it was given assurance that the conditions underlying the training of nurses could be met, e.g. the provision of adequate resources and tutorial service.

The Briggs report was kept 'in abeyance' gathering dust for nine years before the enactment of the Nurses, Midwives and Health Visitors Act 1979, which substantially reflected the report's recommendations. From the discussion that prevailed at the time it was clear, because of the major and far-reaching demands of the Briggs recommendations in terms of finance and manpower, that this long-term delay was inevitable.

The foregoing reports identified the need for and/or precipitated a need for change in nursing. Even through their intentions were sound, the structures that were developed as a result of their recommendations were not always satisfactory. For example, there was inadequate financing at basic and post-basic level; studentship continued relatively unchanged, i.e. learners continued to be used as a major part of the nursing workforce; there was inadequate supervision of learners; counselling and support services remained relatively undeveloped; there was heavy reliance on nursing assistants; untrained staff were left in charge of wards; and there was still employment of agency staff.

The Salmon recommendations, even though they were intended to effect positive change, particularly in relation to the management of nursing, were perceived to undermine and erode the authority and autonomy of the ward sister. This authority and autonomy, when removed from the ward sister, led to the development of other posts, e.g. domestic supervisor, catering manager, etc. Salmon assumed that this would free the ward sister from domestic tasks and enable her to focus on the nursing management of the ward. In retrospect this so called freedom has its limitations. Failure of a domestic to carry out their job satisfactorily results in the ward sister having to refer the matter elsewhere as opposed to dealing with it directly, which leads to less freedom and more time wasted. This is further exacerbated today with the 'contracting out' of domestic and catering services.

In this context, an article by Tolliday (1972) further discussed nurses' uncertainty about their role and concluded: 'When ward sisters insist that the wards are "theirs" and that they must therefore have control over everything which goes on in them, they are interpreted as requiring exactly the opposite, that they want, in fact, to be accountable for all duties required to be carried out in the wards' (para. 8, p. 53). This point on the erosion of nurses' authority was emphasized at a seminar (RCN, 1982) some 16 years later, when it was recommended: 'At each level, accountability should be matched by the necessary authority to control the environment of care'. Associated with the recommendation was 'concern over the extent to which the ward sister's role had been eroded' (para. 4, p. 2).

The EEC Nursing Directives (1977/89) together with the Nurses, Midwives and Health Visitors Act 1979, Nurses, Midwives and Health Visitors Rules Approval Order 1983, and Project 2000 (1986) were a serious attempt through legislation and education to initiate change and control practice in the structures within which nursing education and nursing practice take place, enabling improvement of standards and quality of care and enhancement of job satisfaction for nurses.

Many things affect the way nurses perform their role, e.g. education and training, leadership and support services, the nature and extent of their responsibility and accountability, the extent of their authority and autonomy, their career prospects and job satisfaction. Benne and Bennis (1959), in an article relating to the role 'conflict' and role 'confusion' of the professional nurse, recognized that there were many points of confusion and conflict, including the hospital/organization in which nurses worked, colleagues and nurses' own expectations, which could adversely affect the way nurses were motivated, gained job satisfaction and approached their job.

CONTROLLING PRACTICE

The nursing care of the patient today makes great demands on nurses' knowledge and skills especially if the care given is to be competent, efficient and effective. To meet these goals nurses must have the necessary authority to manage the ward and control nurses' practice. There is considerable discussion within the profession regarding the issues of nurses' authority (this will be fully explored in Chapter 6); the question asked is whether nurses have the requisite authority and autonomy to manage their wards effectively. Opinion is divided. A view expressed by an officer of the nursing statutory body and supported by a representative of the nursing professional body is, 'Limitations of nurses' authority and autonomy are their own doing and is due to their lack of confidence and knowledge. Nurses' authority and autonomy are potentially present; but traditional attitudes of professional managers and doctors prevent their use'. If this view is accurate, inevitably it will lead to constraints and stunting of any new initiatives and developments in nursing, if nurses themselves lack the confidence to take them forward, by failing to use key elements of their role.

When discussing a new professional structure for nursing the RCN (1983) commented: 'The possession of clinical skills and expertise cannot ensure that high standards of clinical care are maintained: they must be accompanied by the authority to manage the clinical environment. The expert experienced ward sister should be given greater autonomy within her own clinical area' (para. 2.5, p. 6). Some interesting points arise from this statement which in practice might create problems for senior nurse managers. For example, how could optimal authority and autonomy be measured? How could the different levels of 'expert experienced' be defined and subsequently graded as 'greater' or 'lesser'?

There is a contrast in the expressed opinions of the RCN: the officer claims nurses have the requisite authority but do not use it; the 1983 document is seeking 'greater' authority for nurses. With the assumption that authority and autonomy can be graded to suit the level of decision to be made by the ward sister/staff nurse, will this guarantee that these will be used effectively in practice? This poses major educational questions for managers and nurse educationists in the way professional nurses are prepared for their role.

Tradition is said to be the basis of many of the ills of the nursing profession. However, tradition itself is good, if it serves to maintain what is good practice and helps nurture and develop new initiatives. Traditional attitudes that become entrenched and prevent acceptance or even consideration of anything new can totally disable any organization. Professor Baroness McFarlane (1983), when commenting on the nursing service, made interesting observations on the professional/traditional accepted view of nursing:

> If one looks at the cost of the nursing service, the nursing needed to give a basic level of care and to maintain the demands of technological support to the medical function, is it unrealistic to expect the nursing service also to support informed personalised care and that feeling of being cared for that aids the patient in sickness? If it is unrealistic then we should cease

to call nursing 'nursing'. Our new name should denote the role of the technical side and our training should reflect the objectives and competencies and tasks rather than the role.

(Para. 3, p. 18)

I see no significant change. For example, we still have not defined what we really mean by 'nursing'. This is coupled with the fact that the profession continues to be swamped and diluted with carers, no doubt all with high ideals and motivation, but with preparation for so demanding a role that is, to say the least, minimal and fragmented. This situation is comparable to the current moves by government to change the face of the teaching profession in primary schools, by employing mothers to assist with the teaching at what is considered the most important level of education. Teachers think this is expediency at the expense of children's education. The Professional Teachers Association at their annual conference (July 1993) totally rejected this government proposal. However, the nursing profession has over the decades perpetuated the situation regarding the employment of nursing auxiliaries/ care assistants/support workers, without real questioning or censure, to carry out what is perceived by many to be the most important level of patient care.

The lack of definition of nursing brings in its wake problems that relate to 'boundary issues' of both the basic and extended nurses' roles. These are lack of clarity and definition of the role, lack of preparation for the role, increased professional accountability particularly related to nurses' 'extended' role and nurses' responsibility and accountability. These factors are perceived by nurses themselves and by nurse managers and doctors as well as the professional body (RCN) not to be in accord with their authority and autonomy. In this context a statement of the RCN (1988) acknowledges:

Nurses in each era have assumed general acceptance of where the boundaries of nursing lie, even though these boundaries have shifted constantly. The debate has focused on particular activities or procedures regarded as being 'non-nursing duties' or part of the 'extended role of the nurse'. 'Non-nursing' duties are felt to require less skill than that of a nurse, and have therefore been delegated to auxiliaries, or domestic or similar workers. Activities regarded as constituting an 'extended role' for nurses are often those inherited from doctors, who do not want that kind of repetitious work, or consider it does not require medical skills.

(Para. 1, p. 3)

What is the validity of this in practice? More importantly, what is its reality? In essence, have nurses over the years passively accepted work that doctors think is beneath their role? Or have doctors realized that nurses are fellow professionals, with skills and knowledge that enable them to carry out these tasks? Have nurses become excited and provided themselves with an extended role that in effect is neither valid nor practicable insofar as it embodies those tasks which doctors regard as menial and which disable them in providing a quality service? These are serious matters and merit investigation and verification if nursing is ever to become a profession in its own right. This indecisiveness of the nurses' role is expessed by the ICN (1965) and the EEC (1977), who state that this is largely due to 'the complexity and lack of definition of nurses' work'.

The changing role of the nurse, particularly the front-line nurse, ward sister and staff nurse, has been a topic of extended discussion for many years, a topic which will no doubt gather momentum as nursing progresses into the next century. This change in role has many roots and is exemplified in 'guidelines' developed by nursing professional bodies, notably the Royal College of Nursing (1988) and the Department of Health, Nursing Division (1989). Why this emphasis on the changing role of the nurse? What are the reasons underlying this heightened discussion on nurses' role?

To attempt to answer these questions one must seriously consider change in society as a whole, including greater public awareness in general, and in particular an improved awareness by patients/clients of their rights, which in part can be attributed to access to information, media enlightenment and more emphasis placed on health matters. In addition, changing health care needs together with advances in medicine, science and technology will call for changes in the way nurses meet these new demands and initiatives. This will affect how nurses are trained and educated in the context of how they meet their new demands and responsibilities. It will ultimately mean that nurses who do not update their skills and knowledge will have diminished or even non-existent career prospects. This is correct and proper. Many ward sisters (67%, $n=21$) and staff nurses (76%, $n=74$) interviewed in the study, especially those who had been qualified for 5–30 years, had undertaken little or no postgraduate training. This must change for the profession to have integrity and offer quality care. Nurses cannot assume that they enter the profession 'for life' and rely on basic skills, some acquired years previously. Perhaps nurses have brought the conflicts and dilemmas upon themselves by not addressing their own inadequacies. During the study, many ward sisters (39%) and staff nurses (53%) said they felt 'inadequate' in addressing the many onerous duties of their role, especially the demanding commitment to the teaching, assessment and counselling of nurses. Staff nurses particularly emphasized the increased demands of their 'additional' facilitator/mentor role.

This point was acknowledged by the report (DoH Nursing Division, 1989) which reflected concern on the lack of nurses' professional development and some nurses' lack of concern about their own professional development: 'It must be a matter of concern that today's nurses do not routinely have facilities for period refreshment, apart from the mandatory requirements for midwives. Nor indeed do they always recognise the need to update skills imparted to them during education, possibly two or three decades ago' (para. 43, p. 23).

In light of the foregoing, how can postregistration nurses be expected, on the principles of adjusting their scope of practice (UKCC, 1992b), to comply with the injunction that they 'Must endeavour always to achieve, maintain and develop knowledge, skill and competence to respond to the needs and interests of the patient or client', and 'must honestly acknowledge any limits of personal knowledge and skill and remedy and deficits' (paras 9.2/9.3, p. 6). To bring into focus nurses' responsibility and associated accountability in ensuring their own competence and professional development, there is a need to look at the way postregistration nurses are trained and developed.

PROBLEMS OF EDUCATION

There is clearly a need to move from the premise and tradition that once nurses are trained and registered this guarantees their competence throughout their career. Preregistration education only certifies competence at the time of registration. Postregistration education and development should be continuous throughout the entire period of nurses' employment.

The Judge report (1985), one of the major recent documents to appraise the education of nurses, explores many educational problems that act as impediments to the progression of the nursing profession into the next century:

> The startlingly high proportion of students of nursing must 'learn' from a dangerously small number of qualified nurses, many of whom have been only a short time in post, and who are unevenly distributed throughout the system; in practice, the central error of treating learners as an integral part of the workforce (though recent requirements and conditions imposed by the nursing statutory bodies, limits this practice, at least in theory) . . . proportionately large numbers of students working on the wards severely constrain the effective supervision which they need and the sympathetic support which they deserve.
>
> *(Paras 1.4–1.11, pp. 8–10)*

Arising from this exploration of lacunae in the training and development of nurses, a similar situation arose in my own study, which found an acknowledged shortage of experienced and appropriately skilled professional nurses to supervise, teach and counsel learners; no nurse learner was regarded in a supernumerary role, they were an integral part of the ward workforce.

In discussions with colleagues and in the wake of Project 2000, many say this problem should have been resolved. However, there continue to be many shortcomings in the way learners are developed. For example, on wards where learners are supernumerary, the staff are often too busy to teach, develop or supervise them, and they stand around doing nothing, whereas those considered to be an integral part of the ward team carry out many tasks without supervision, teaching or support. These areas need to be addressed urgently.

DILEMMAS OF THE NURSES' ROLE

The dilemmas for professional nurses and nurse managers, from the foregoing analysis which provides the backcloth to this book, identify some of the difficulties inherent in nurses' future role and can be summarized thus: attempting to maintain an effective nursing service in an environment that presents a vagueness of role, functions and professional parameters; and not knowing the area of legitimate clinical freedom and practice. Paramount is the notion that the authority, responsibility, accountability, autonomy and development of nurses do not match the demands of their role, functions and expectations and mitigate against nurses meeting the needs and demands of patients. In essence, their imprecise role is relatively unproductive and unmeaningful in meeting the demands placed upon them, in their ability to meet those demands, and more importantly in their continuing security and job satisfaction. The roots of the problem thus unfolded are many, complex and often firmly entrenched in the tradition of the nursing profession and the development of nurses' professionalism over many decades.

Many reports, papers and laws already discussed have attempted to influence change with limited effect. However, even though some change has met with disapproval and apathy, it cannot be disputed that substantial progress has been made in achieving some of the cited objectives, notably in the education and development of nurses and patient care.

Change makes many demands on staff and is alarming for some who have difficulty in facing the reality in respect of the organization or the profession in which they practise. Change, especially change of a major nature, has marked effects on the behaviour of nurses who often are not suitably prepared for change and its effects. Therefore, nurses' proper preparation, at all levels of the profession, must be a priority of management, ensuring as far as possible nurses' ability to cope with change and achieve success for themselves, their patients and the organization.

This necessitates a clearly defined education/orientation programme to enable staff to learn new behaviours often while adjusting and adapting to a new role; most importantly, this often necessitates the unlearning of some existing behaviours in relation to their existing role. In this situation, to obviate staff problems and insecurity, the potential and/or actual problems associated with the role changes must be made known. In this context a report of the National Foundation for Educational Research (Leonard and Jowett, 1990), based on a study of six ENB pilot schemes in preregistration nurse education, makes a relevant point which should be heeded by those introducing change: 'There was unanimity across all schemes that the process of implementation had confirmed that the introduction of change is an extremely long term and time-consuming process, that innovation cannot be achieved overnight, especially if it is to last. A continuous process of staff development has to be instigated as a first priority' (para. 5, p. 14). The problems and their perceived causes, which have implications for practice and the future role of the nursing profession, will be discussed in subsequent chapters.

2	# The study – rationale, design and methodology: profile of district health authorities

RATIONALE

From the survey of the literature and the related research on roles in general and in particular the role of the nurse, some pertinent views expressed provided triggers for the rationale, theoretical framework and methodology of the proposed study.

The literature reviewed included that of Anderson (1973), Cang *et al.*, (1981), Hardy and Conway (1978), Kramer (1966, 1974), Pembrey (1980), Williams (1969), the UKCC (1984) and government reports and papers. The information thus presented enabled a more lucid and realistic focusing on the problems that were ultimately investigated.

The ideas of Mintzberg (1968, 1970, 1971, 1973), Patton (1978) and Whitmore (1971, 1973) greatly influenced the adoption of the methodology. The work of these authors facilitated the structuring and ultimate design of instruments used, i.e. the structured interview schedule and non-participant observation schedule. Whitmore's interview schedule on work study was adapted and subsequently formed the basis for the observation schedule used in the study.

The study in essence was qualitative and exploratory. The general aims of the study were to establish the main behaviours, duties, tasks and responsibilities for which professional nurses are accountable, together with appraising the extent of their authority and autonomy to manage their wards and care for their patients; to identify a curriculum appropriate to meeting the professional/educational needs of professional nurses; and to assess the relationship between the manifest, assumed and extant aspect of the nurses' role, i.e. the prescribed, assumed and actual behaviours of nurses. The particular aims and objectives of the study focused on investigating and clarifying the present role of the professional nurse.

Hypotheses

The study was based on the following hypotheses:

1. There exist differing perspectives on the nature (elements and orientation) of the role of the professional nurse, ward sister/charge nurse and staff nurse, as perceived by professional nurses themselves, nurse managers, doctors and the nursing professional and statutory bodies, in the context of nurses' manifest (prescribed/agreed), assumed (by nurses and significant others) and actual role.
2. There exist disparity and imbalance between the authority (power to make decisions relevant to the job) and the autonomy (freedom to expedite those decisions without censure) to care for their patients and to manage their wards professionally, i.e. to meet patients' needs effectively and efficiently.
3. The educational/professional development of professional nurses is inadequate and/or inappropriate to enable them to meet the requirements and demands of their prescribed/agreed role.

Formal approval

Following informal exploratory talks with two district health authorities, permission to pursue the fieldwork was provisionally agreed and a formal research proposal was submitted for approval to the University of Newcastle upon Tyne. The proposal was accepted, unqualified. Subsequently, a formal approach was made to the district health authorities to pursue the study. This was agreed.

The study was carefully introduced and explained to staff at every level of the organization, with a request for their co-operation. As patients were to form part of the sample, permission was obtained from the chairpersons of the medical ethical committees of both district health authorities. Formal feedback was given to the respective medical ethical committees and senior nurse managers every six months on the progress of the research. All staff and patients included in the final sample were seen and had the proposals of the study discussed individually with the researcher. The nature and purpose of the research was explained and their participation in the study was invited. All nursing staff agreed. Two doctors were unable to participate 'because of their commitments'. Two patients preferred 'not to take part' for undisclosed reasons.

Pre-pilot study

Following agreement to pursue the study, a pre-pilot study was conducted (Table 2.1) to sample the views and opinions of staff and patients in the clinical specialities in order to establish criteria for the pilot study.

Table 2.1 Constitution of sample of 30 for pre-pilot study

Grade/profession	Clinical speciality			Total (n)
	Acute medical	Acute surgical	Longstay	
Ward sister/charge nurse	2	2	2	6
Staff nurse	2	1	0	3
Enrolled nurse	1	0	1	2
Nursing student[a]				10
House officer	0	2	0	2
Consultant	1	0	1	2
Patient	1	2	2	5

[a] Interviewed during study block.

Thirty interviews were conducted. All were tape recorded. The average time taken for interviews with nurses and doctors was 45 minutes. The average time taken for each patient interview was 25 minutes.

Staff and patients invited to participate in the study were randomly selected from staff rosters and ward lists, given explanation and invited to participate. All volunteered. The method used for interviews included the use of open-ended questions, which reflected the general dimensions of the role of the professional nurse together with patients' perceptions of their needs during their stay in hospital.

The pre-pilot study proved to be of considerable value in establishing a framework for the instruments that were subsequently piloted. The rich and varied responses obtained enabled the subsequent development of the instruments to be focused in the pilot study.

Pilot study

Selection of staff and patients was done on the basis of convenience following initial invitation and explanation (Table 2.2). All volunteered. It was agreed by the supervisors of the research to exclude nursing students and enrolled nurses, and focus the study on the role of the registered nurse. The sample for the pilot study was constructed as follows.

Pilot of instruments

Structured interview schedule
For further information, see Chapters 4 and 5, Tables 4.1 and 5.1 and Appendices A and B. The comments received from interviewees following piloting of the structured interview schedule were most favourable. In the main, respondents underlined the 'clarity' and 'reality' of the instrument and

Table 2.2 Constitution of sample of 11 for pilot study of structured interview schedule and non-participant observation schedule for different clinical specialities

Grade/profession	Acute medical			Acute surgical			Longstay		
	Inter-view	Obser-vation	n	Inter-view	Obser-vation	n	Inter-view	Obser-vation	n
Ward sister/charge nurse	1	1	1	1	1	1	1	1	1
Staff nurse	1	1	1	2	2	2	1	1	1
Nurse manager (deputy)	1	0	1	1	0	1	0	0	0
House officer	1	0	1	0	0	0	0	0	0
Registrar	0	0	0	1	0	1	0	0	0
Total	0	0	4	0	0	5	0	0	2

indicated that the time for each interview (approximately 45 minutes) did not interfere with their duties. Nurse managers and doctors also regarded the time taken as satisfactory and adequate for discussion of the topics presented.

Non-participant observation schedule
The schedule (Appendix A) was tested by two independent nurse managers and the researcher. The results were favourable in terms of the validity and reliability of the instrument. However, the readiness of the instrument to record data in an effective and efficient way posed a problem that was subsequently obviated by further testing and modification of its framework.

Patients' interview schedule
The schedule (Chapter 7, Table 7.5) was readily accepted by patients in terms of its time (15 minutes) and content.

COMMENT

From the pilot study, the central role of the professional nurse was essentially perceived (by nurses and doctors) as 'caring', 'nursing' or 'clinical'. The status (authority, autonomy) of the nurse was seen by all nurses as being central to the proper (professional) performance of the nurses' role. The authority and autonomy of the nurse were agreed as prerequisites for enabling decisions to be made in the management of the ward and the provision of a quality, high standard of nursing service to the patients. In their absence, the nurses' role was perceived to be substantially 'muted' and 'passive'.

The preparation of nurses for their potential role (ward sister, charge nurse and staff nurse) was seen to be especially lacking in social skills, e.g.

counselling and interpersonal competencies, together with the 'practice skills' required of professional nurses, relating to ward management and ward administration. The ongoing education, training and development of the nurse was emphasized as a priority for ensuring sound practice.

The 'nursing process' was viewed by many nurses and doctors to have many limitations, including duplicating patients' medical history and too much paperwork, which consequently reduced nurses' time with their patients. Some nurses additionally said: 'little information was obtained from care plans; they did not deal with patients as individuals, but as numbers, and patients' needs were not properly identified and evaluated'. Nurses and doctors summarized the nursing process as 'a lot of information which was irrelevant' together with 'a duplication of medical records'.

Following a satisfactory conclusion to the piloting of instruments it was agreed by the university supervisors to go ahead with the final phase of the study.

THE MAIN SAMPLE

Framework and constitution

The framework on which the structured interview schedules were based reflected the extensive research on roles in general, and the role of the professional nurse in particular, together with informal information and the information obtained through the pre-pilot and pilot studies, substantially based on the job descriptions (Appendix B) provided by both district health authorities. Job descriptions were described by nurse management as being 'crammed with everything', 'very general' and 'historically defined', i.e. based on the ideas of the Salmon Report (1966) and varying in time from their initial development, i.e. 3–10 years.

Extracts (nurses' key obligations) from the *Code of Professional Conduct for Nurses, Midwives and Health Visitors* (UKCC, 1984) were included in the design of questions, to reflect professional nurses' responsibilities and their accountability for their clinical practice.

A non-random, convenience sample using volunteer patients, nurses, nurse managers and doctors as well as representative officers of the statutory and professional bodies (Table 2.3) was used to facilitate the exploratory discussions which formed the main phase of the study.

The central aspect of the methodology was influenced by the ideas of many authorities, especially those of Patton, Mintzberg and Whitmore, which were agreed to be particularly useful in the general design of the instruments and which formed the framework of the preferred methodology. In this respect, the ideas of Patton (1978) on qualitative interviewing and observational methods were agreed, by supervisors, to be particularly useful in the context of data collection. In qualitative interviewing, Patton addressed three approaches,

Table 2.3 Constitution of main sample for different clinical specialities in two district
health authorities (DHA)

Grade/profession	Acute medical DHA 1	Acute medical DHA 2	Acute surgical DHA 1	Acute surgical DHA 2	Longstay DHA 1	Longstay DHA 2	Number interviewed DHA 1	Number interviewed DHA 2	Number observed DHA 1	Number observed DHA 2
Ward sister/charge nurse	3	3	6	5	2	2	11	10	3	3
Staff nurse	16	16	20	17	2	3	38	36	8	8
Unit nurse manager	1	1	1	1	1	1	3	3	0	0
Consultant	1	1	3	3	2	1	6	5	0	0
Registrar	1	1	1	2	1	0	3	3	0	0
Senior house officer	0	1	0	2	0	1	0	4	0	0
House officer	2	1	2	2	0	1	4	4	0	0
Total	24	24	33	32	8	9	65	65	11	11

Also interviewed: the senior nurse manager from each DHA, one officer from each
statutory and professional body (ENB, UKCC, RCN) and a 25% sample of patients
from each observed ward.

namely 'informal conversational', 'general interview guide approach' and
'standardized open-ended interview'. The last approach was used in the study
as the most appropriate means of exploring nurses' role.

'Essentially, the standardized open-ended interview comprises a set of
questions worded and arranged with the intention of taking each interviewee
through the same sequence and asking each the same questions with the same
words'. In practice, the open-ended interview enabled data to be collected that
were systematic and thorough for each interviewee. This approach minimized
variation in the questions posed to interviewees. The interview schedule used
in the study contained more than 50% open-ended questions and closely
followed the principles outlined by Patton.

Patton acknowledged four approaches to observational methods along the
continuum of observation, originally defined by Junker (1960), which
included 'complete participant', 'participant as observer', 'observer as
participant' and 'complete observer'. The approach used in this study was that
of 'complete observer'. Activities were completely public. Staff of the wards
observed were fully informed of the situation and their confidence and co-
operation was secured.

The intention of the observational aspect of the study was to describe the
setting that was observed, the activities (macro) that took place in the
particular setting and the people who participated in those activities. This
approach was in accordance with Patton's theory. The observation schedule
used in the study was used to record the activities that took place, including a

description of the physical setting in which the activities took place, the direct quotations of nurses and the observers' reflections about the personal meaning, interpretation and significance of what took place.

In addition to Patton's ideas, it seemed appropriate that Mintzberg's (1970) views on structured observation as 'a method that couples the flexibility of open-ended observation with the discipline of seeking certain types of structured data' would enhance the collection of observation data. In this respect, 'in addition to categorizing events, the researcher is able to record detailed information on important incidents, enabling the researcher to observe and question intensively, to be systematic and to develop theory inductively'.

Whitmore (1971, 1973) described 'activity sampling' as 'a method which can be adopted for work measurement in order to determine a true standard for performing a task, often at a defined level of performance'. The method is based on observations of the activity made either at random or at regularly spaced intervals, i.e. 'fixed interval sampling'. After discussions with Whitmore, the activities schedule designed by him was, with his approval, adapted, adjusted and tested as a means of recording the observational data (Appendix A).

In the study, major activities (behaviours), e.g. managerial, administrative, clinical, educational (nurses and patients), communication (nurses, doctors, patients and time on telephone, giving and receiving information), direct supervision of nurses, time spent on waiting, time spent on official rest periods and time spent on walking between activities were observed and recorded at 1.5-minute intervals for three 2-hour periods. The schedule included an additional column to include miscellaneous activities observed, i.e. those not already identified.

This method enabled a 'snapshot' to be taken of the nurses' job, though, because of the limited time and the small number of nurses observed, this could be used only as a general index of nurses' behaviours, while additionally serving as a guide to the nurses' perspective of their job, stated during interview. The major behaviours observed were previously identified through the pre-pilot and pilot studies and the nurses' job descriptions. The method used, in additional to recording the number of observed activities, enabled a full profile to be recorded of the ward at the time of observation.

An interview manual was kept to ensure that any required amplification/clarification of questions was constant. The structured interviews that were used in the study had the following categories: general information; ward profile; staff profile; operational definitions; duties (functions); responsibilities; caring; patients' needs; and education, training and development.

The observation of nurses produced a description of the setting observed, a record of activities (behaviours) that took place and descriptive information about what nurses did, to whom they spoke and what they said (direct quotations). This facilitated the recording of the observer's own reactions and reflections on the meaning of what occurred and what was said; i.e. by being close to the situation, the observer was able to 'move beyond the selective perceptions of other professionals'.

Each nurse was observed for 6 hours, three 2-hour consecutive sessions (Table 2.4), with recording of observations at 1.5-minute intervals at different times of the professional nurses' working day, e.g. early morning, mid-morning and late afternoon.

Table 2.4 Observations of nurses

| | Clinical speciality | | | | |
Grade of nurses	Acute medical	Acute surgical	Longstay	Hours observed	Number of observations
Ward sister/charge nurse	2	2	2	36	1440
Staff nurse	6	8	2	96	3840
Total	8	10	4	132	5280

Night staff were not included in the sample, largely because of the inadequate numbers of trained nurses on night duty with limited back-up staff, and the constraints of time on their availability.

Twenty-two nurses were observed (for details see Table 2.4). A total of 240 observations for each nurse were recorded. In total 5280 observations were recorded. By using a variety of sources and resources, i.e. interviews, observation and checking relevant documentation associated with the nurses' job, despite the limitations of the sample size, it was hoped to increase the validity and reliability of the data. The data from the pre-pilot and pilot studies enabled the totality of the situation in the main study to be more readily understood, allowing for different dimensions and elements of the nurses' role, without imposing pre-existing expectations other than any bias acknowledged by the researcher, because of previous experience.

Definition of terms and concepts

For ease of readership, terms and concepts used in the study deemed to be effective focuses for the behaviours explored were defined as follows.

Administrative   Any activity that is related to ward routine, but which is not deemed to be immediate to the patients' condition and/or care, e.g. preparation of reports and hospital returns.

Authority   'The rightful (legitimate) power to fulfil a charge' (Batey and Lewis, 1982).

Autonomy   'Freedom to make discretionary and binding de-
                    cisions consistent with one's scope of practice and
                    freedom to act on those decisions' (Batey and Lewis,
                    1982).

Behaviour   'The action or actions of some living thing'
                    (McDougall, 1969).

Clinical   Any activity that relates to the patient's condition.

Communication   Any activity that relates to the giving and receiving
                    of information, e.g. directions, reports, discussion or
                    informal conversation between nurses, doctors,
                    patients, relatives or others, professional or
                    non-professional.

Direct supervision The direct overseeing of nurses in their performance
                    of clinical, managerial or administrative tasks.

Duties   The tasks (work) that are related to the job of the
                    professional nurse, deemed by nurse management to
                    be appropriate to their role.

Education   Any activity that relates to the formal teaching/
                    instruction of nurses or the formal (intentional)
                    informing of patients on matters relating to their
                    health (health education) and to their care.

Function   'The activities assigned to the incumbent of a social
                    status' (*On Theoretical Sociology* by Robert K.
                    Merton. © 1967 by Robert K. Merton. Used with
                    the permission of The Free Press, a division of
                    Macmillan, Inc.)

Macro elements   Macro/major elements are activities elicited through
                    discussion with nurses and doctors, information
                    from the job descriptions of professional nurses,
                    elements identified by the pre-pilot and pilot studies
                    prevalent in the job of the nurse (not minutiae).

Managerial   Any activity that relates to the general management
                    of the ward, including the management of nursing
                    staff and the ensuring/enabling of patient services.

Miscellaneous   Included as an extra column in the observation
                    schedule to record events (behaviours) occurring,
                    which were not included in the listed behaviours.

Needs   'Requirements for the maintenance of personal
                    wellbeing'. (Reproduced from Kraegel *et al.*, 1972,
                    with permission from Mosby-Year Book, Inc.)

Patient dependency 'The amount of care patients require to meet their
                    needs at a given time' (Goldstone, 1983). Goldstone
                    described three categories of dependency:

1. High-dependency patients. This category denotes 'maximum care; the patient is totally dependent upon the nursing staff for his care'.
2. Intermediate-dependency patients. This category denotes 'average amount of care required; the patient is able to provide some care without assistance'.
3. Low-dependency patients. This category denotes 'virtual self-care; the patient is quite independent for his personal care'.

Perceive	'Process by which individuals give meaning to their environment' (Nord, 1972).
Professional nurse	Registered nurse, ward sister/charge nurse/staff nurse.
Responsibility	'A charge for which one is answerable' (Batey and Lewis, 1982).
Resting	Time taken for official meal breaks.
Role	'The part/s played, and the tasks performed by individuals together with the services they are entitled to receive from other people in recognition of their contributions' (Banton, 1968).
Senior nurse manager	A senior, experienced nurse, with particular responsibility for the overall organization of nursing services of a hospital/s within a district health authority.
Task	'A specific job of work' (Brown, 1971).
Time on telephone	Includes time involved in giving and receiving of information in relation to ward management, patients and nursing staff.
Unit nurse manager	A senior, experienced nurse, with responsibility for a particular clinical speciality, usually two or more wards and/or departments.
Waiting	Inactivity between tasks.
Walking	Walking to and from nurses' station/office, before commencing and/or completing any activity.

Even through both district health authorities had discrete titles for the nursing officers at middle and senior management levels, for the purpose of this study the titles 'unit nurse manager' and 'senior nurse manager' were used. Both district health authorities used the term 'geriatric' for longstay care of the elderly wards.

Following from the satisfactory completion of the pre-pilot and pilot studies, preparation for the final phase of the study was made. The organization of the main sample was designed and developed from the findings of the above studies. Timetables, appointments and schedules were prepared for the main study.

Constitution of sample

Twenty wards were included in the study. A total of 135 structured interviews were conducted with staff (registered nurses, nurse managers and doctors); 81 interviews were conducted with patients. In addition interviews were conducted with officers of the two nursing statutory bodies and the nursing professional body. Twenty-two nurses were observed.

Profile of participating district health authorities

The study was conducted in two district health authorities within the Northern Regional Health Authority (Table 2.5). Six hospitals and 20 wards,

Table 2.5 Mix of specialities in two district health authorities (DHA)

Description	Acute medical	Acute surgical	Longstay
DHA 1			
Male medical	1		
Male surgical		1	
Male orthopaedic		1	
Male geriatric			1
Gynaecology		1	
Female medical	2		
Female surgical		2	
Female geriatric			1
Total	3	5	2
DHA 2			
Male/female medical	1		
Male/female surgical		1	
Male medical	1		
Male surgical		1	
Male geriatric			1
Gynaecology		1	
Female medical	1		
Female surgical		1	
Female orthopaedic		1	
Female geriatric			1
Total	3	5	2

including six acute medical wards, ten acute surgical wards and four longstay (geriatric) wards were used for the fieldwork.

Ward profile

The average number of patients on the acute medical, acute surgical and longstay wards were 21, 23 and 19, respectively.

Patient dependency on medical wards was perceived by nurses, nurse managers and doctors to be 'high' (above average); on surgical wards patient dependency was perceived to fluctuate between 'high' and 'intermediate' (average care). On longstay wards patient dependency was perceived to be persistently high; many patients required individual care, which often necessitated the involvement of two members of staff (usually nursing auxiliaries).

The average length of patient stay on acute medical and surgical wards was stated to be 14 days and 6 days, respectively. The majority of patients on longstay wards were rarely discharged into the community.

Staff profile

In the main, the status of the sample was female (Table 2.6).

Table 2.6 Status of sample

Grade/profession	Male	Female	Total
Ward sister/charge nurse	3	18	21
Staff nurse	1	73	74
Unit nurse manager	1	5	6
Senior nurse manager	1	1	2
Doctor	26	3	29
Officer of statutory body	1	1	2
Officer of professional body	0	1	1
Patient	36	45	81
Total	69	147	216

Even though there was no intention deliberately to stratify the sample proportionately and/or disproportionately, other than to include representative grades and professionals for each speciality (Table 2.7), the final numbers of staff interviewed were reasonably representative of the total establishment, e.g. ward sister/charge nurse (25%), staff nurse (33%) and doctors (25%).

Table 2.7 Staff establishment whole-time equivalents

	District health authority	
Grade of staff	1	2
Ward sister/charge nurse	73.00	97.00
Staff nurse	151.00	158.84
Enrolled nurse	117.00	154.71
Nursing student (not extranumerary)	96.00	99.00
Nursing auxiliary	155.00	117.58
Ward clerk	12.00	3.00
Doctor[a]	58.00	83.00

[a] Included consultants, registrars, senior house officers and house officers.

The mix of skills and grades of staff on medical and surgical wards differed little. Longstay wards in the main relied on nursing auxiliaries to carry out patient care. Most wards were dependent on nursing students for direct patient care. (There were no nursing students on longstay wards.) Also, even though ward clerks were employed, this was done on a part-time basis. The practice in the main was for wards to share clerical assistance.

Many nurses perceived there to be a 'heavy' workload (in excess of normal/expected) and inadequate staffing levels, particularly a lack of registered and experienced nurses. Both district health authorities used agency nurses. However, one district recruited its own registered nurses. This was enabled by the policy of the district, which ensured the employment of all registered nurses as bank nurses, for whom jobs were not available following their registration.

The age on appointment to post for ward sisters was on average over 30 years. The age on appointment to post of staff nurses was under 23 years (Table 2.8).

A total of 72 nurses, including eight ward sisters and 64 staff nurses, held one professional qualification. Eight ward sisters held two qualifications; four held three qualifications and one held four qualifications. Seven staff nurses held two qualifications and three held three qualifications (Table 2.9).

COMMENT

The continuity of professional nursing staff on wards in both district health authorities was good, though the districts had a policy of rotating professional nurses, especially staff nurses, between wards as part of their 'staff development' programme. Also, ward sisters were encouraged to rotate from day duty to night duty and vice versa. Senior nurse managers explained the

Table 2.8 Age on appointment to present post in two district health authorities (DHA)

Age (years)	Acute medical		Acute surgical		Longstay		Total	
	DHA 1	DHA 2	DHA 1	DHA 2	DHA 1	DHA 2	DHA 1	DHA 2
Ward sister/charge nurse ($n=21$)								
Under 23	0	0	0	0	0	0	0	0
23–26	1	1	1	0	0	0	2	1
27–30	1	1	2	2	1	1	4	4
Over 30	1	1	3	3	1	1	5	5
Staff nurse ($n=74$)								
Under 23	10	11	8	6	0	0	18	17
23–26	0	3	6	3	0	0	6	6
27–30	3	0	2	1	0	1	5	2
Over 30	3	2	4	7	2	2	9	11

Table 2.9 Professional qualifications in two district health authorities (DHA)

Qualification	DHA 1			DHA 2			n
	Medical	Surgical	Longstay	Medical	Surgical	Longstay	
Enrolled nurse	0	0	0	1	1	1	3
Registered general nurse	16	20	2	16	17	3	74
Registered mental nurse	2	0	0	0	1	1	4
Registered midwife	0	0	1	0	0	0	1
Family planning certificate	0	0	0	0	1	0	1
Orthopaedic nursing certificate	0	0	0	0	2	0	2
Diploma in professional studies in nursing	0	0	1	0	0	0	1
City & Guilds 998	0	0	0	0	1	0	1

philosophy underlying the rotation of professional nurses in the following terms.

District Health Authority 1: 'Staff nurses move annually for their development, though this is a cause of concern to them and to doctors; this causes a break-up of the existing, established ward team and requires further adjustment to meet the clinical and skill needs of the nurse. People get buried on night duty and lose their clinical and managerial skills, they become out of touch with current change'.

District Health Authority 2: 'The intention is to develop staff, particularly in managerial skills. There are different needs and demands to different specialities'.

The policy of staff rotation was perceived by senior nurse management as useful; many nurses, especially staff nurses, together with many doctors and some ward sisters, viewed this practice with suspicion and unease. Their main complaints related to the 'unsettling' effects of breaking up the ward team, and the effects of this practice on staff, many of whom felt 'uncomfortable' and 'stressed' by this rotation and expressed some difficulty in adjusting to a new clinical speciality and environment that was not of their choosing. Doctors' views concurred with the views expressed on the rotation-related problems, and underlined the particular organizational/clinical problems, particularly noting the dissolution and subsequent time wasted on re-establishing a good working relationship and understanding with key nurses.

Perceptions of professionals (doctors and nurses) of the ethos of the clinical environment

During interviews many nurses and doctors underlined 'differences' in their perception of their clinical specialities. These perceived differences, on discussion with nurses and nurse managers, included not only the more obvious differences of workload and patient dependency but also the perceptions of staff on the 'stability' and 'orderliness' of the clinical specialities. For example, it was often stated (particularly by ward sisters and to some extent by staff nurses and doctors) that the acute surgical wards were 'ordered', 'stable' and quite 'predictable' insofar as admission of patients was fairly regular and predictable (arranged admissions); operations in the main were predetermined, including a likely date for the discharge of patients. However, despite these 'regularities', the turnover rate for patients was rapid (many spending little time in hospital), which produced an additionally heavy workload, especially for nurses. Many ward sisters and doctors commented on the limited number of beds, which prevented them from coping professionally and caused the transfer of patients who were nearing discharge to other wards. This caused additional problems for nurses who were responsible for transfer arrangements, as they were sometimes abused by patients and their relatives.

In contrast, the medical speciality was perceived to be less 'stable', less 'ordered' and less 'predictable', especially in the context of patient admissions. Many patients were confined to bed and required constant and additional vigilance.

The perceived 'disruptiveness' and unpredictability of medical wards was often stated to be due to the frequent occurrence in elderly patients of stroke and cardiac arrest, as well as to their frequent mental and emotional deterioration. Medical wards were perceived to be especially emotionally stressful, not only from the additional demands of the elderly patients, but also from the necessity of having to cope with younger patients following attempted suicide.

Nurses stated that there was an acute shortage of medical beds, a view substantiated by nurse managers. This often necessitated transfer of patients to other wards.

The longstay speciality was described as 'regular', 'predictable' and of a very 'demanding' nature for nurses, physically and emotionally, with many patients requiring constant support, vigilance and help. Many longstay patients remained in hospital for many months and/or years. What better evidence do we need that an integrated community care programme, now enacted, is long overdue to enable patients to be nursed in their own homes if they so wish?

In summary, most wards perceived a shortage of staff which prevented nurses providing the standard of care they would wish. Many nurses and doctors acknowledged a lack of certain facilities, e.g. hoists and toilet facilities as well as a shortage of monitoring equipment and syringes, which they said sometimes necessitated borrowing from other wards. From the information given, many staff nurses lacked substantial clinical, administrative and managerial experience to equip them to meet their onerous responsibilities of managing their wards and ensuring patient care and, additionally, adopting a 'mentor/facilitator' role, which was required by nursing management.

Despite these shortcomings, the activities of nurses who were observed, together with the accounts that were given by other professionals during interviews, served as a general though useful indicator to what was ultimately revealed in the findings of the commitment of nurses, which was unquestioned, ensuring, sometimes against the odds, the care of their patients. Many staff nurses in the acute medical and surgical specialities had limited experience in post, even though they were frequently left in charge and required to undertake full responsibility for the management of their ward, including ensuring the care of their patients together with the leadership, supervision and teaching of nursing students and/or other staff including nursing auxiliaries. ('Nursing auxiliary' was the title used in both health authorities.)

Eighteen staff nurses had 1–3 years' postregistration experience and 21 staff nurses had under one year's experience (Table 2.9).

Tables 2.8 and 2.9 illustrate the implications for the local (hospital) nursing service which, irrespective of the goodwill, enthusiasm and industry of these staff nurses, could potentially undermine the viability and the implementation of the envisaged educational reforms. Some of the initial disclosures, especially those relating to the diverse nature of each clinical speciality with its demands and shortcomings, together with the concerns expressed by many professionals on workload, responsibilities, authority and autonomy, professional development and standards of care have clear implications for the implementation of Project 2000 (UKCC, 1986) if they continue unresolved. The full nature and the implications of the findings will be discussed in subsequent chapters.

Findings of the study: résumé of the evidence and supporting data

In this chapter the main findings of the study and supporting data are discussed with reference to other relevant research. How did nurses perceive their role? How did other professionals perceive the role of the professional nurse? Did nurses meet their professional statutory obligations to themselves, to their patients and to nursing management? How did patients perceive that their needs were met? How confident were nurses at giving a professional service? Was the education of nurses adequate in helping them to cope with change – technological, social and educational?

The findings in some instances were ambivalent, sometimes gave rise to alarm and on occasion to undeniable apathy of the nursing profession to resolve some longstanding problems relating to their role.

TESTING OF VARIABLES

The chi-squared test was used as a test of association for all variables (for details of responses by nurses and other professionals, see Chapters 4, 5 and Appendices A, B and C). Variables were tested for trends in confidence levels. Many of the variables tested showed reasonable confidence levels, varying from 85% to 99.5%. Variables within these parameters had frequencies that were equally distributed for all professionals in both district health authorities and in all clinical specialities. However, on analysis, some variables showed differences between the observed and expected frequencies. For example, a higher number of observed than expected frequencies was recorded in both the medical and surgical specialities. No such variation was noted in the longstay speciality.

On discussion with statisticians and supervisors who were consulted on the design of the instruments and the nature of the sample, it was proposed that this distribution was probably a product of chance, due largely to a difference of perception, i.e. differing perceptions of nurses and other professionals to the questions asked and/or to the differing nature of the clinical environment in which they worked. In this respect, surgical wards were perceived by many to be 'more ordered and predictable' in their nature and their activities, whereas medical wards were perceived to be 'less ordered and predictable'. Also, it was agreed that the identified variations on chi squared analysis could be distortions due to the relatively small though professionally representative sample, which limited full statistical analysis. Variables that showed reasonable levels of confidence on initial testing, i.e. in excess of 85%, were further tested using the chi-squared statistic by combining columns (1 and 2, 3 and 4). This approach showed no further change in the initial confidence levels recorded.

The results thus obtained, even though not statistically significant, are interesting and useful when examined in the context of the rating by nurses, who often demonstrated their inability to meet many of their responsibilities.

In addition to testing for trends in confidence levels, the variables used in the patient interview schedules were also tested. The results on analysis showed high trends in confidence levels varying between 95% and 99.5%, demonstrating how well or otherwise patients perceived that their needs were met (see Chapter 7 and Appendix E).

MAIN FINDINGS

The following is a résumé of the main findings.

Nurses' role

The role of the nurse, i.e. the part played by the ward sister and staff nurse, was explored by examining the perceptions of nurses themselves and other professionals' perceptions of their role by exploration of nurses' prescribed/defined duties and responsibilities, their perceived authority and autonomy and their state of readiness for their role (Chapters 4, 5 and 6). Essentially, nurses perceived their basic role as one of 'caring' and 'nursing'.

Virtually in complete contrast and with some conviction nurse managers perceived the role of nurses, especially ward sisters, to be 'managerially' and 'administratively' orientated. The staff nurses' role was seen to be more 'nursing' and 'teaching' orientated. On discussion with nurses and doctors, this paradox produced a dilemma for many ward sisters and staff nurses, which they said adversely affected their motivation and job satisfaction for a role which lacked proper preparation in skills and knowledge, stating:

Currently you are flung into the new role with little or no preparation relating to the particular problems of ward management, new developments and change. At first you tend to panic. There should be a gradual phasing and acquisition of skills to meet staff nurses' responsibilities in the final year of studentship. Staff nurses should be given three months' training on qualifying; they should be supported, not crushed.

In practice, the observation of nurses' behaviours revealed a multidimensional role containing components of management, much administration and a nursing element, more for staff nurses than ward sisters, together with a teaching component, often difficult to expedite. Many ward sisters and staff nurses said they had little if any time for teaching, with few staff to teach due to staff shortages, because when students and auxiliaries were on duty they were often too busy delivering nursing care and they themselves were overloaded with administrative tasks and caring for their patients.

Ward sisters perceived their role to consist of 70% managerial/administrative behaviour, 20% direct patient care and 10% teaching (nurses and patients). Staff nurses perceived their role to consist of 30% managerial/administrative behaviour, 45% direct patient care and 25% teaching, mainly of nursing students. Little difference in the reality of the nurses' role was perceived by nurses themselves, nurse managers, doctors and officers of the statutory and professional bodies. The role of ward sister and staff nurse in terms of the job content were virtually identical, with staff nurses regularly (daily) in charge of the ward in the sisters' absence, often with little support.

Nurses in the main perceived that they had the requisite authority to manage their wards and to care for their patients despite stated evidence to the contrary, e.g. their acknowledged inability to influence resources in an appreciable, effective way, and their difficulty in ensuring professional standards of care. Nurses subjectively seemed to be saying that their status and role, i.e. 'ward manager', gave them the requisite authority irrespective of the reality of the constraints, e.g. staff and material resources. Nurses agreed that their lack of autonomy, insofar as they were unable to make key decisions on patient care, was an acknowledged impediment to their professional practice. Some ward sisters stated: 'Doctors interfered with and altered established nursing care regimes, and some would not accept their advice on the care of patients'.

Many nurses acknowledged impediments to their professional development, including the lack of resources, finance and staffing, which they perceived to be difficult, if not impossible to ensure, because of their lack of authority.

From the evidence, there was a distinct lack of support, guidance and counselling for nurses at all levels. These shortcomings emphasized by recently (1–3 years) registered nurses, made them 'feel vulnerable'. Nurses indicated their 'unease' about being given a role, often 'thrown in at the deep end', for which they had not been prepared emotionally, occupationally or organizationally (not being aware of their role in the organization as a whole). In this context it was often stated by staff nurses that their job description accompanied their letter of appointment and not the application form.

Most importantly, many ward sisters (20%, $n=4$) and staff nurses (50%, $n=37$), many of whom had been employed by that district for a number of years, had not undertaken further training and updating (for details, see Chapter 9).

Many of the role-inherent problems acknowledged in the study are not new. Evidence can be found in *Some effects of exposure to employing bureaucracies on the role conceptions and role deprivation of neophite collegiate nurses* (Kramer, 1966), *Reality Shock: Why Nurses Leave Nursing* (Kramer, 1974), *The Role of the Nurse* (Anderson, 1973), *Role Theory: Perspectives for Health Professionals* (Hardy and Conway, 1978), *Improving Health Care Management: Organization Development and Organization Change* (Wieland, 1981) and *Boundaries of Nursing* (RCN, 1988). The role of the nurse and some of its major components will be fully discussed in subsequent chapters.

Standard and quality of care

Most nurses directly related the lack of resources to their inability to ensure proper standards and quality of patient care, i.e. the provision of care at an acceptable professional level where the needs of their patients were met unconditionally. Doctors, nurse managers and officers of the statutory and professional bodies supported this view. This was also emphasized in recent Audit Commission reports (1991, para. 29; 1992, para. 24). In practice, much of the direct 'hands-on' care was given by nursing students (average 80%) and nursing auxiliaries (average 90%). This was especially obvious on longstay wards.

The responses of many ward sisters (34%, $n=7$) and some staff nurses (25%, $n=18$) indicated that the objective (stated criteria) evaluation of patient care did not feature to a great extent in their job; this perception was substantiated by some (33%, $n=2$) unit nurse managers and many doctors (79%, $n=24$).

The majority of ward sisters (86%) and staff nurses (90%) said they could not care for their patients professionally, i.e. especially ensuring the safety and wellbeing of their patients. This acknowledgement by nurses was also substantiated by some unit nurse managers (33%), senior nurse managers and the majority of doctors (83%) (Table 3.1). This finding is echoed generally in many other reports and documents spanning virtually 60 years but still continues to plague the profession.

For example, the Royal Commission on the National Health Service (Merrison, 1979), when referring to standards of care, stated:

Table 3.1 Perceptions of nurses and other professionals of nurses' ability to care for patients professionally. All clinical specialities and district health authorities 1 and 2 included

	Response (%)			
Grade/profession	Yes	Yes (qualified)	No	n
Ward sister/charge nurse	14	0	86	21
Staff nurse	3	7	90	74
Nurse manager	0	67	33	6
Senior nurse manager	0	0	100	2
Doctor	17	0	83	29
Statutory body officer	0	0	100	2
Professional body officer	0	0	100	1

Much evidence had been received by its Committee expressing concern about declining standards of nursing care which was often attributed to the structural change arising from the Salmon and Mayston Committees' recommendations [Mayston, 1969] and their alleged tendency to withdraw good clinical nurses into administration. The evidence submitted indicated that the main areas of risk in hospitals related to untrained staff left in charge of wards, inadequate supervision of learners, neglect of basic nursing routines and the employment of agency staff.

(Para. 13.5, p. 185)

The report concluded that: 'These are serious matters and there is no doubt that nurses are under pressure in many places, and services to patients suffer' (para. 13.6, p. 185).

A report of the Royal College of Nursing (1984) implied difficulty in establishing what was meant by 'standards of care' and stated:

Standards of care is a difficult concept to discuss simply because there are so many ways to measure standards. But when nurses themselves say that through staff shortages they are no longer able to give a level of care that, as professionals, they know the patient requires, this is cause for real concern.

(Para. 5, p. 34)

Further information relating to problems in delivering safe, effective care together with the absence of personalized, person-related care are discussed by Aiken (1981) and in a report of the Department of Health, Nursing Division (1989).

It was agreed by senior nurse managers that many impediments, including heavy workload (a workload that could not reasonably be met by nurses), staffing problems and the lack of nurses' own professional development prevented them from ensuring high standards of care and safe standards of practice. Concern was expressed by 34% of ward sisters and 25% of staff nurses that, to a great extent, they were unable to evaluate objectively (by use of agreed criteria) the care given to their patients. This view was substantiated by two unit nurse managers and many (80%, $n = 24$) doctors. In fact the evaluation of care was largely done subjectively.

Both district health authorities used Monitor (Goldstone, 1983) once every 18 months as 'an audit of quality'. During periods of observed nurses' behaviour it was evident that on many occasions nurses were unable to care for their patients as they would have wished. However, given the constraints of acknowledged staff shortages and lack of facilities, e.g. wash basins, toilet facilities and sometimes equipment needed for basic nursing/medical procedures, nurses were always seen to care for their patients to their utmost ability. There was some difference of opinion among nurse managers regarding the validity of this situation, especially relating to ward staffing; they claimed that often staffing was adequate but the way staff were utilized was ineffective. This and other identified evidence on standards of care for whatever reason continue unresolved.

Patients' needs

For further details, see Chapter 7 and Appendix E. A report of the Department of Health (1989) stated: 'The essence of nursing will always be the organized and professional response to individual need' (para. 1, p. 17). How does this view compare with the findings of this research on the reality of the nurses' role meeting patients' needs? In light of the previously identified evidence on falling standards of care and nurses' admission of certain inadequacies in meeting their responsibilities, how did patients perceive that their needs were met? 'Nursing standards are how well an individual nurse meets an individual patient's needs' (RCN, 1981; para. 3, p. 2).

A number of patients (38%, $n = 32$) perceived that some of their 'physical' needs and many of their 'emotional' needs were badly met, especially identifying those of explanation, fear reduction and advice about their health, together with a lack of privacy, dignity, confidentiality, rest and sleep. Many patients also stated that much of their stress was contributed to by many of these shortcomings, central to which were the conspicuous lack of information, fear of operation/anaesthetic and worry about their personal health.

During observation periods the main elements of patients' dissatisfaction were lack of sleep, e.g. being awakened at 6.30 AM, given a cup of tea and asked to go back to sleep again; lack of dignity, such as inadequate toilet facilities and not being given a bowl to wash after bedpans, thin curtains between beds, nurses asking about 'waterworks' and 'bowels' in loud voices; lack of confidentiality; having their clinical condition discussed in loud voices at the foot of the bed by the ward team; and lack of independence (nurses doing too much for patients).

In the main, younger patients (20–40 year age group) commented more openly and vigorously on the inadequacies of the service than did middle-aged and elderly patients who, with few exceptions, accepted the situation. Female patients in their comments were more anxious about home and family matters and the lack of advice and information than were male patients.

Some impediments acknowledged by nurses, which prevented them meeting patients' needs, included the geography of many wards, which were large and inconvenient (Nightingale type), the lack of trained experienced staff, inadequate outmoded equipment and facilities, workload, lack of time and ward/hospital practices, e.g. waking patients at 6.30 AM. There is much evidence supporting these findings. Some reports propose ways of solving these problems, such as those of Revans (1964), Briggs (1972), Merrison (1979), DHSS (1979), RCN (1984), Visser (1984) and the Audit Commission (1991, 1992).

Role of the patient

After interviews with nurses, nurse managers and doctors, and from the observed behaviour of nurses (six ward sisters and 16 staff nurses were observed in three clinical settings, each for a period of three 2-hour periods, observations being made at 1.50-minute intervals), it was clear that there was little involvement of patients in their care programme, nor indeed in their health education. This lack of involvement of patients was seen, on the basis of some nurses' responses, to have its roots in expediency, which they often related to 'inadequate time' and 'staffing problems', nurses finding it 'easier and quicker' not to involve patients in their care. To highlight the problem ironically, one nurse manager stated 'the patient does not have a role'.

During periods of observed nurses' behaviour, patients in the main had a passive role. Nurses' interactions with patients, especially in the form of communication, were few even when they were carrying out personal care. Patients' requests, e.g. for pain relief and personal toilet, were sometimes delayed or ignored without explanation.

Recent publications (RCN, 1988; DoH Nursing Division, 1989; Audit Commission, 1991, 1992; UKCC, 1992a, 1992b) emphasize many of the problems outlined and suggest solutions.

Manpower and other resources

Many nurses were 'unhappy' about the lack of other resources and/or the lack of their quality, e.g. wheelchairs, hoists, sphygmomanometers and infusion stands, a situation which they often regarded to be time consuming, in that it often necessitated having to borrow equipment, even in emergency situations.

Additional lack of and/or inadequacy of rest rooms, recreational facilities and rooms where patients could discuss matters of a confidential nature with staff were perceived by nurses and doctors to be highly unsatisfactory and caused much frustration for patients and staff. Further information that amplifies the issue of resources can be found in recent Audit Commission reports (1991, 1992). The 1991 report found 'Evidence collected for the study suggest that some resources within nursing could be used more efficiently to release funds for investment in clinical training, and professional and managerial training for nurses', and 'Many nurses still spend over a quarter of their time on clerical and housekeeping tasks. A minority of wards systematically collect data on nursing workload and fewer still put the resulting information to good use. Bank nurses are frequently booked regardless of predicted workload' (paras 4/1, pp. 1/2). In the same context the 1992 report found 'A need to bring responsibility for care and control of ward resources much closer together and a need for greater clarity in management roles and relationships, particularly those of ward sisters and their immediate superiors' (para. 57, pp. 27/28).

The information from my own study reveals that ward sisters (56%) and staff nurses (89%) were unable to ensure the resourcing of their wards, to the extent they felt was essential, due to their perceived lack of authority and autonomy. The irony of the situation thus portrayed focuses on nurses' accountability to local nursing management (their employer) as well as to their nursing statutory body (the UKCC), to ensure patients are cared for professionally and there are always the proper resources (over which, regrettably, the nurses have little authority and less autonomy). In fact, unit nurse managers and senior nurse managers emphasized that the provision and the matching of resources to the workload of the ward was the sole responsibility of the unit nurse manager. In practice, ward sisters and staff nurses (when in charge of the ward) could only inform and advise but not insist on what they deemed to be the proper resourcing of their wards. A statement by one senior nurse manager focused the problem with the statement: 'The manpower resourcing of wards is done on a convenience basis'.

Many of the points were made evident during periods of nurses' observed behaviours. It became clear that there were staff shortages but the utilization of nurses' skills was not efficient. For example, time was spent doing clerical work that could have been done by a ward clerk.

One particular example of the lack of authority of the staff nurse was found on a busy surgical ward where seven patients were being prepared for theatre. The ward staff at the time consisted of one staff nurse, one enrolled nurse and a nursing auxiliary. The policy of the hospital correctly insisted that each patient be escorted to and from theatre by a trained nurse. The staff nurse in charge, who was under considerable pressure, frequently requested additional help, sometimes to enable her to take a short rest break. None of the requests were met.

The evidence, advice and elucidation on resources and the problems of inadequate resourcing are in abundance (Taylor, 1962; Kraegel *et al.*, 1972; Merrison, 1979; RCN, 1984; Price Waterhouse, 1987; URCC, 1989; DoH Nursing Division, 1989; UKCC, 1992a, 1992b).

Responsibilities and accountability

The responsibilities that were addressed in the study (Chapters 5 and 6) were substantially based on the job description of the nurse and the UKCC *Code of Professional Conduct* (1984), which details professional accountability. There were 28 responsibilities addressed: clinical (7), managerial (12) and educational (9). The three categories of responsibilities were agreed by nurses and other professionals to have many limitations in their realization. For example, key responsibilities, including acknowledging and managing the workload and pressure on colleagues and subordinates, were 'seldom' met.

Most ward sisters (66.6%) and many staff nurses (59%) stated they had difficulty in 'completely' safeguarding the wellbeing of their patients, ensuring high standards of care (57%, 69%) and giving information to patients and relatives (43%, 16%). Communication with patients together with ensuring their safety and wellbeing, which they deemed essential to ensure a quality service, was impossible to achieve due to lack of time and pressure of workload.

Unit nurse managers were divided in their responses on how well trained nurses met their responsibilities. It was indicated by 33% that nurses had particular difficulty in ensuring the respect of patients' customs (according to the *Code of Professional Conduct*, para. 6) and safe standards of practice. It was emphasized by 67% that there were marked limitations in nurses' ensuring the adequacy of resources. In practice, they agreed, this was their responsibility. Many (50%) stated that nurses had difficulty regulating/managing the workload and pressure on colleagues and subordinates. They also said that nurses rarely, if at all, counselled staff, and that the feasibility of ward sisters and staff nurses ensuring their professional competence together with its associated personal and professional development was limited.

Senior nurse managers had marked reservations on the feasibility of nurses being able to fulfil many of their responsibilities clinically, managerially and educationally.

Many doctors stated marked reservations about nurses meeting virtually all of the listed responsibilities, particularly emphasizing those of safeguarding the wellbeing of patients, which 48% said could not be met, ensuring high standards of care (62%), safe standards of practice (65%) and respecting the confidential information of patients (24%). Many rated some managerial responsibilities as 'seldom and/or never met', including nurses' ability to regulate the workload of colleagues (38%) and subordinates (34%) and to acknowledge/adjust the pressure on colleagues (38%) and subordinates (34%).

Officers of the nursing statutory and professional bodies were pessimistic in their responses as to professional nurses meeting certain key clinical responsibilities, notably those of safeguarding the wellbeing of patients, ensuring high standards of care and safe standards of practice and meeting, to a reasonable extent, the needs for respect of patients' customs. Some managerial and educational responsibilities were also perceived not to be satisfactorily met, including dealing with workload and pressure on colleagues and subordinates, ensuring proper resources, ensuring their personal competence and professional development and effecting the health education of their patients. In this context they perceived the non-use of authority and autonomy by some nurses, which they attributed to traditional reasons, e.g. nurses' perceived subordinate role to other professionals, nurses' lack of assertiveness and their inability to make decisions, contributed to nurses' inability to meet their statutory/professional obligations.

During periods of nurses' observed behaviour many nurses found difficulty in regulating their workload and pressure on colleagues. There was little evidence of direct supervision of staff and communication with patients. On discussion with nurses following periods of observed behaviour, they commented: 'I can be aware of pressures on staff but can't always do anything to relieve them, especially if they are work-based'; 'I cannot always carry out medical instructions. Sometimes what doctors say is not physically possible, e.g. mobility of patients may require two nurses; without proper staffing this is not possible'. These are typical of the comments made by nurses in both districts, often supported by doctors and nurse managers. As a postscript to these findings it is interesting to note that some of the issues discussed were identified some 60 years ago. The Lancet Commission on Nursing (Earl of Crawford and Balcarres, 1932) found: 'many nurses in training objected to the hurried work necessitated by insufficient staffing; others complained of being given excessive responsibility before receiving adequate instruction' (Appendix iv, p. 179).

The many issues of nurses' responsibility/accountability have been discussed in-depth over many years (Briggs, 1972; Merrison, 1979; Aiken, 1981; RCN, 1988; UKCC, 1989, 1992a, 1992b).

Authority and autonomy

In the light of the former findings (for details see Chapter 6 and Tables 6.1, 6.2 and 6.3) and nurses' perceived or actual inability to meet many of their responsibilities, as a direct result breaching their code of professional conduct, were they hampered by a lack of authority and autonomy?

Many ward sisters (67%) and staff nurses (77%) acknowledged having the requisite authority to manage their wards and care for their patients. Many ward sisters (91%) and staff nurses (92%) perceived constraints to their autonomy. In contrast, unit nurse managers, senior nurse managers and doctors perceived marked limitations to nurses having both the requisite authority and autonomy.

Despite many nurses' responses to the contrary, and observation of nurses' work, it was evident that nurses did not participate in decision making on nursing policy and in fact had little control, other than to request the proper resourcing of their wards. As a direct effect of these shortcomings in their job, nurses could not ensure to their satisfaction the care and wellbeing of their patients. Paradoxically, many stated on interview that they had the requisite authority to ensure the proper care of their patients, whereas in reality the following comments illustrate the situation: 'There is little choice in nursing practice as policy is decided elsewhere by the Nursing Procedures Committee and nursing management; there is little flexibility to alter what is decided' and 'I can inform the unit nurse manager about patient dependency levels, which is done three times a day, but I cannot ensure staffing levels to meet patients' needs'. Why this anomaly? Why this apparent confusion? The answer probably lies in the difference in nurses' perception and interpretation of what constitutes the reality of nurses' 'objective' and 'subjective' authority. This conflict is discussed in Chapter 6.

The following authors help to clarify the reality and importance of nurses' authority and autonomy: Mayeroff (1971), Cang et al. (1981), Hardy and Conway (1978), Rowbottom and Billis (1987), the RCN (1988) and the Audit Commission (1991).

Nurses' stress

Not unexpectedly, and in light of the many difficulties, problems and conflicts already attributed by nurses to their role (see Chapter 8), many nurses perceived their role to have a stress level in excess of that which they expected and which could be readily tolerated. For example, many ward sisters (71%) said their role was 'very stressful'. The majority of staff nurses (90%) acknowledged an excessive (more than usual) physically and emotionally disabling level of stress.

Somewhat surprisingly (despite the much publicized evidence), unit nurse managers stated there was little if any 'additional' stress, other than that which was expected, in the job of the nurse. This view was not upheld by senior nurse managers who underlined 'appreciable levels of stress' in the job of ward sisters and staff nurses, which they unequivocally attributed to the shortage of resources and the nature and demands of ward management, the care of patients and the demands on nurses. Many doctors perceived the nurses' role to be 'very stressful', due to its continuing demands, lack of overt support and a counselling service and sometimes (associated with recently registered nurses) a lack of training together with a lack of the requisite authority to do their jobs with confidence.

Recently registered nurses (1–3 years) stated that they experienced a lack of support in their job and said that one of the main worries was their inability to cope with doctors' ward rounds, planned and unplanned. The direct effects of stress included 'unease', 'disillusionment', 'unhappiness', 'apathy' and low morale, which they said led to the frequently repeated 'lack of job satisfaction'. These findings gave rise to much concern among nurses, a concern which from the evidence was perceived by nurses as not being taken seriously by the profession. For example, neither district which took part in the study employed a system of diagnosis, support, prevention or alleviation of nurses' stress. However, the initiative of one ward sister produced a system of support and counselling for ward nurses. The system operated anonymously, i.e. the recipient was known only to the 'counsellor' of their choice. The ward sister when interviewed said the system was very effective insofar as nurses could confidentially discuss their problems and, should these be of a serious nature, the nurse could be referred to the appropriate agencies. At national level the RCN employs 2.5 counsellors for a membership of 500 000 nurses. Nurses, when asked how they coped with their stress, gave many answers, including: 'have a drink', 'try to forget about it', 'have a good cry', 'talk with friends', 'have a bath' and 'read a book', all of which they acknowledged were expedients, some having inherent dangers!

Nurses' stress, its causes, prevention and management are well documented in the works of Revans (1964), Briggs (1972), Hardy and Conway (1978), Marshall (1980), Wieland (1981), Hingley et al. (1984), Hingley and Cooper (1986) and indeed as far back as the report of The Lancet Commission (Earl of Crawford and Balcarres, 1932). Sadly, according to the nurses interviewed and the evidence obtained, all were apparently ignored or unnoticed!

Transfer of patients

Many nurses, especially ward sisters (60%), indicated their disapproval and frustration at the common practice of transferring patients to other wards, many on the eve of being discharged home.

Both medical and surgical wards were used for the interchange of patients, an occurrence that in the view of many nurses and doctors fell short of good practice and, for many reasons, caused nurses much stress and inconvenience, as well as being a potential source of danger for patients. Ward sisters and staff nurses emphasized that this practice was time consuming in its entirety, because of the arrangements which were required to be made prior to the patient's transfer. They were concerned at the clinical and practice implications associated with this common occurrence, which included lack of nurses' knowledge of patients' needs, particularly their treatment and customs; lack of nurses suitably skilled to cope with any probable emergencies associated with the patient transferred, e.g. nurses working on gynaecological wards might not be adept in the skills of coping with cardiac arrest, stroke and respiratory arrest; conversely, nurses working on medical wards might not be conversant with current gynaecological procedures and practices.

On a more personal note the effect on the patient is very distressing; they are often in tears, frightened and disorientated as they have to adjust to new staff, patients and ward routines.

Equally distressing are the effects of the transfer of patients on nurses, who suffer verbal abuse by patients and their relatives and discouragement because of lack of job satisfaction in not seeing their patients discharged home fit and well.

Senior nurse managers of both districts, when commenting on this practice, said 'the practice is unavoidable due to the shortage of beds, medical and surgical'. One hospital had an estimated shortage of thirty medical beds.

This practice did little to reassure patients and strengthen the continuity of their care. Some of these points are indirectly dealt with in the reports of the Audit Commission (1991, 1992).

Employment of agency nurses

Ward sisters expressed their 'unease' at the regular practice of employing agency/bank nurses, trained and untrained, wrongly in their view, 'to bolster and fill the gaps brought about by inadequate ward staffing levels'. Many (81%) underlined the shortcomings of this policy insofar as, far from enabling the care of patients, it often constituted a potential danger to these patients, because of the lack of knowledge and skills of the nurses thus employed, and their frequent inability to meet the specialist needs of the patients for whom they were caring. Ward sisters and staff nurses often said that this arrangement was also unfair on the agency/bank nurses, because they were frequently sent to a different ward every day; they were unable to get to know their patients and/or build up relationships with ward staff or patients.

Nurses and doctors questioned the safety and the economics of this practice, the financing of which they stated 'could be employed more beneficially, if spent employing permanent nurses'. However, the employment of agency nurses has a parallel in medicine identified during interview by some doctors (25%), especially consultants, who stated that the practice of employing locum doctors was regular and posed similar problems for fulltime doctors as for their nursing colleagues, i.e. there was a lack of commitment by some of these doctors to the hospital and their patients.

Nurses and doctors equally complained about the fact that agency/bank staff for nursing and medicine were paid more than regular staff and were also paid for overtime. The views of Merrison (1979) on the employment of agency staff, though ignored, are clear: 'The evidence given to the Commission, expressing concern about declining standards of nursing care, one of the "areas of risk" in hospitals, was the employment of agency staff' (para. 13.5, p. 185). Other publications discuss some of the problems relating to the employment of agency/bank nurses (RCN, 1988; Audit Commission, 1991, 1992).

Staffing of longstay (geriatric) wards

It was evident in the longstay wards studied that there was a substantial reliance on nursing auxiliaries to ensure the care of patients, with few trained nurses and no nursing students on the staff.

On these wards there was an inordinately heavy workload, a need for much individual patient care and a high dependency rate. During the periods of observation there was no doubt that the elderly, often infirm patients could have benefited from the presence of more professional nursing staff, even though the nursing auxiliaries on these wards were part of what was stated to be 'a stable, permanent workforce' who, from observation, were committed to the care of their patients.

The implication of these findings and from discussions with some nurses and doctors is that elderly longstay patients do not require skilled professional expertise. This is a view not supported by an officer of the RCN, who said 'We are very concerned about the general situation that is highlighted in the lack of care of the elderly and infirm in hospitals'. From observation and discussion with nurses, it was concluded that one longstay ward in particular was impoverished in both manpower and equipment. When commenting on the care of infirm old people in the NHS, the Merrison (1979) report stated:

> In any plans for the care of infirm old people in the NHS nurses must play the most important part: they are the only category of caring staff essential when active treatment is no longer possible. Recruiting and retaining the nurses will present an increasing problem. This is one of the most demanding branches of nursing, calling for personal qualities and skills of a high order.
>
> *(Para. 6.36, p. 65)*

Rotation of nurses

Both district health authorities had a policy of rotation, where registered nurses were moved to a different ward, usually on an annual basis. As a direct result of this policy, many nurses (sisters, 55% and staff nurses, 50%) voiced their concern at the break-up of the ward team to which they had become accustomed. They said they found this experience 'stressful and unsettling'.

Some staff nurses (27%) did not welcome the idea of being moved on an *ad hoc* basis from wards which were perceived by nurse managers at a given time to be 'quiet', to assist or take charge of another ward on a temporary basis (normally during a shift). Many doctors (40%) stated that the practice broke the continuity of the ward team and they were 'unhappy' about it.

Senior nurse managers agreed the practice of rotating staff was 'not liked by nurses and doctors; but it was necessary to enable staff development by exposing nurses to different needs and different demands in other clinical specialties'. Other reasons given to support or rationalize this policy included: 'to give nurse management greater flexibility'; 'staff get buried on nights and lose their clinical and managerial skills'; and 'staff, especially those on night duty, are often out of touch with current change'.

Job satisfaction: expressed satisfaction and dissatisfaction of nurses with their grading

At the time of the study (1988–89) *A Guide to the Clinical Grading Structure* (Nursing and Midwifery Staff Negotiating Council, 1988) was published for staff representatives and others involved in its implementation. Of the 21 ward sisters interviewed, all were 'happy' with their new grade.

The majority (67%) of staff nurses interviewed were 'satisfied' with their grade; of these, 28 were graded 'D' and 21 'E'. Four staff nurses said their grade was 'acceptable', but they were 'not happy' (two Ds and two Es). However, some (28%) staff nurses said they were 'dissatisfied' with their grade (15 Ds and six Es).

Staff nurses who were 'not happy' and/or 'dissatisfied' with their grade included in their reasons: 'excess responsibility' which included often deputizing for the ward sister; extent of experience and expertise together with the nature and length of service to the hospital; and the 'complexity' of their role with which they had to cope, frequently having to work unsupervised. Staff nurses who were 'unhappy' with their grading varied in their time since qualifying from 6 months to 25 years. Those who were 'unhappy' and/or 'dissatisfied' with their new grade had 1–36 years' hospital service. It is difficult to establish the rationale by which decisions on nurses' grading were made. It was stated by an officer of the Royal College of Nursing during interview that 'many authorities were relatively unprepared, essentially because of the absence of objective criteria to expedite the process of grading, which subsequently proved to be of enormous difficulty for nurses'. The view stated, based on feedback from nurses and their own interpretation of this, was that nurse managers were caught with their 'trousers down'; wholly 'unprepared'; common guidelines had not been agreed by management and staff; discussion with staff had been 'immensely variable' and 'patchy'; and 'the whole exercise had not been handled sensitively'.

Education, training and professional development

Most nurses perceived their basic nurse training in terms of preparing them for their potential and predetermined nursing and caring role (Chapter 9). They said the last six months did not focus on preparation for their immediate future role. In this respect, many expressed concern at being disadvantaged by lack of knowledge and skills of 'the doing' aspect of the job, including ward routine, management and administration, which they were expected to be in command of immediately on becoming registered nurses. Of the 21 ward sisters interviewed, 81% perceived their basic training to be 'unsatisfactory' and 'too narrow' insofar as it was 'too theoretically' orientated, and that it failed to prepare them for their future role of staff nurse. Ward sisters (19%) perceived their training to be 'satisfactory' in that it provided a 'sound approach' to basic nursing, linked theory with practice, and provided them with 'some insight' into their future role.

Of the 74 staff nurses interviewed, 57% said their training was 'inadequate', 'unrealistic', 'narrow' in its nature, 'did not encourage/ensure their participation' (it was substantially prescribed and didactic) and failed to provide a 'realistic' preparation for the role of staff nurse. Ten (14%) staff nurses said their training was 'too narrow' and 'too theoretical' in that it failed to link the theory taught with the practical care of the patient. Twenty-two (30%) said their training was 'good' and/or 'satisfactory' and they 'enjoyed' it, in that it provided relationships between theory and practice, 'nurses were able to relate to their teachers' and they were 'free to express their views' and were 'encouraged to challenge statements made'.

Four ward sisters had not undertaken further training since qualifying; 17 had undertaken various short courses on counselling, assessing (English National Board Certificate 998), and/or teaching skills (City and Guilds Certificate 730); and, additionally, five had undertaken some form of first-line management training.

Of the 74 staff nurses, 32 had not undertaken further training since qualifying; 25 had attended short courses ranging from one and a half to two days in length and 17 had undertaken training of one week or slightly more. Of the entire number of staff nurses interviewed, only nine had undertaken a first-line management course.

Finally, other important findings on nurses' education, training and development indicate that many nurses perceived difficulty ensuring their own professional knowledge, skills and updating. This they attributed to inadequate or unrealistic staffing levels, which prevented them taking time off to attend in-service and external courses, and to obvious limitations associated with attempting to ensure the updating of many staff. Few nurses stated that they undertook courses on their own initiative and in their own time. When asked to amplify this, some said they were 'too tired' to undertake further study, because of their workload and its pressures, and/or they were 'not afforded the opportunity' to undertake further study because of 'the lack of reality of staffing levels'. Many nurses (ward sisters and staff nurses) stated that because of too many demands on their time and too few trained and qualified staff, they could not teach and supervise untrained and unqualified nurses in the way they wished, if at all.

This point is amplified by Judge (1985), who states that 'Many ward sisters have neither the time nor the inclination to provide effective student supervision' (para. 1.7, p. 9). Publications relating to these findings include WHO (1966), Salmon (1986), RCN (1988), DoH Nursing Division (1989), Audit Commission (1991), UKCC (1992a, 1992b).

The findings of this study highlight the many problems which, despite voluminous evidence, continue to plague the profession and demonstrate its inadequacy to come to terms with the reality and challenges of nurses' role now, and to take nurses with integrity into the future.

These problems require urgent solutions if the profession is to provide the service expected and legally demanded, as envisaged in the objectives and philosophy of Project 2000. Or will the lack of finance and the lack of professional development of nurses hamper this initiative?

As a postscript, two vital questions must be addressed: What is the cost, in financial terms, of commissioning, preparing, and publishing, over decades, many official reports? Most importantly, what is the cost, in terms of the service to patients, of the continuing inaction?

These questions in particular and the findings of this study in general will be discussed more fully and some solutions proffered in subsequent chapters.

The job of the nurse: the data as revealed by investigation and analysis

In this chapter the job of the nurse, including its duties and tasks, is discussed. The information was derived from in-depth interviews with nurses (ward sisters, $n=21$; staff nurses, $n=74$) and non-participant observation of a sample of these grades. A four-point scale was used to determine the extent to which behaviours took place. The explored duties were rated on a range as to their realization from 'great extent' to 'little extent'. The following definitions were used:

Great extent: Featured regularly, daily, in job
Fair extent: Featured often, but not daily
Some extent: Featured occasionally, infrequently
Little extent: Featured seldom, if at all

Four categories of behaviours were identified, i.e. clinical (12), managerial (12), administrative (6), and educational (6). Tables 4.1 and 4.2 give the responses of ward sisters and staff nurses. For responses of other professionals, see Appendix C.

COMMENT

The clinical behaviours thus explored demonstrated general agreement by nurses in both districts of their marginal influence in determining nursing policy. There was clear evidence on the extent to which nurses engaged in direct patient care. On interview many nurses said that most of the listed clinical behaviours featured regularly in their job, a perception also acknowledged by nurse managers, though not borne out by the evidence provided by observation. Even though nurses in the main accepted many of

THE JOB OF THE NURSE

Table 4.1 Rating (%) by 21 ward sisters/charge nurses of the extent to which prescribed duties featured in their job

Duty	Great extent	Fair extent	Some extent	Little extent
Clinical (management of patient care)				
1. Determining nursing policy	33.33	28.57	4.76	33.33
2. Identifying patients' needs	90.48	9.52	–	
3. Prescribing nurses' work (in the context of nursing care and medical instructions)	80.95	19.05	–	–
4. Planning nursing care (defining patient-care objectives)	71.43	19.05	9.52	–
5. Delivering nursing care (having direct contact with patients)	38.10	42.86	14.29	4.76
6. Integrating the work of the ward team	80.95	9.52	4.76	4.76
7. Setting nursing standards (ensuring high standards of care)	95.24	4.76	–	–
8. Evaluating nursing care (against defined nursing objectives)	66.67	28.57	4.76	–
9. Fulfilling nurses' legal obligations (drugs, treatment)	90.48	4.76	4.76	–
10. Fulfilling nurses' ethical obligations to patients (confidentiality)	95.24	4.76	–	–
11. Ensuring the independence of patients (ensuring freedom of activity within prescribed levels)	66.67	28.57	4.76	–
12. Other	–	–	–	–
Managerial (general management of ward)				
1. Deciding what work has to be done (establishing goals)	80.95	19.05	–	–
2. Allocating work	61.90	33.33	–	4.76
3. Co-ordinating the work of the ward team	85.71	14.29	–	–
4. Ensuring accountability for work done	85.71	9.53	–	4.76
5. Monitoring the work of nurses	90.48	9.52	–	–
6. Ensuring the adequacy of resources	42.86	42.86	9.52	4.76
7. Organizing resources (matching resources to workload)	66.67	28.57	4.76	–
8. Communicating with ward team	95.24	4.76	–	–
9. Communicating with patients	85.71	14.29	–	–
10. Counselling staff	90.48	–	9.52	–
11. Appraising staff	85.71	14.29	–	–
12. Leading ward team	95.24	4.76	–	–
Administrative (ward routine but not patients' condition)				
1. Ordering ward stock	38.10	33.33	14.28	14.29
2. Checking ward stock	42.86	28.57	23.81	4.76
3. Requisitioning resources	57.14	19.05	14.29	9.52
4. Preparing returns for nursing/hospital management	76.19	14.29	9.52	–
5. Writing reports	85.71	14.29	–	–
6. Arranging meetings (ward policy)	42.86	28.57	14.29	14.29
Educational (teaching, instructing and/or informing)				
1. Induction of trained nurses (new to ward)	80.95	14.29	–	4.76
2. Induction of nursing students (new to ward)	33.33	33.33	28.57	4.76
3. Planning the educational experience of nursing students	33.33	47.62	19.05	–
4. Teaching staff	57.14	28.57	9.52	4.76
5. Teaching patients (health education)	42.86	38.10	–	19.05
6. Counsel staff as appropriate	47.62	28.57	19.05	4.76

Table 4.2 rating (%) by 74 staff nurses of the extent to which prescribed duties featured in their job

Duty	Great extent	Fair extent	Some extent	Little extent
Clinical (management of patient care)				
1. Determining nursing policy	20.27	14.86	13.51	51.35
2. Identifying patients' needs	94.59	5.41	–	–
3. Prescribing nurses' work (in the context of nursing care and medical instructions)	75.68	20.27	4.05	–
4. Planning nursing care (defining patient-care objectives)	82.43	16.22	1.35	–
5. Delivering nursing care (having direct contact with patients)	62.16	33.78	4.05	–
6. Integrating the work of the ward team	60.81	35.14	4.05	–
7. Setting nursing standards (ensuring high standards of care)	82.43	16.22	–	1.35
8. Evaluating nursing care (against defined nursing objectives)	75.68	21.62	2.70	–
9. Fulfilling nurses' legal obligations (drugs, treatment)	95.95	4.05	–	–
10. Fulfilling nurses' ethical obligations to patients (confidentiality)	97.30	2.70	–	–
11. Ensuring the independence of patients (ensuring freedom of activity within prescribed levels)	41.89	51.35	4.05	2.70
12. Other	–	–	–	–
Managerial (general management of ward)				
1. Deciding what work has to be done (establishing goals)	60.81	37.84	1.35	–
2. Allocating work	64.86	33.7	1.35	–
3. Co-ordinating the work of the ward team	56.76	41.89	1.35	–
4. Ensuring accountability for work done	68.92	29.73	–	1.35
5. Monitoring the work of nurses	68.92	25.68	1.35	4.05
6. Ensuring the adequacy of resources	9.46	44.59	25.68	20.27
7. Organizing resources (matching resources to workload)	20.27	44.59	17.57	17.57
8. Communicating with ward team	81.08	16.22	2.70	–
9. Communicating with patients	87.84	12.16	–	–
10. Counselling staff	22.97	33.78	14.86	28.38
11. Appraising staff	28.38	29.72	14.86	27.04
12. Leading ward team	37.84	50.0	9.46	2.70
Administrative (ward routine but not patients' condition)				
1. Ordering ward stock	21.62	40.54	24.32	13.51
2. Checking ward stock	28.38	51.35	16.22	4.05
3. Requisitioning resources	17.57	45.95	24.32	12.16
4. Preparing returns for nursing/hospital management	29.73	45.95	17.57	6.76
5. Writing reports	78.38	17.57	1.35	2.70
6. Arranging meetings (ward policy)	35.62	4.11	15.07	45.21
Educational (teaching, instructing and/or informing)				
1. Induction of trained nurses (new to ward)	44.60	18.92	10.81	25.68
2. Induction of nursing students (new to ward)	77.03	12.16	5.41	5.41
3. Planning the educational experience of nursing students	55.41	25.68	12.16	6.76
4. Teaching staff	41.89	27.03	17.57	13.51
5. Teaching patients (health education)	56.95	30.56	12.50	–
6. Counsel staff as appropriate	31.51	26.03	15.07	27.40

the managerial behaviours listed, this was not substantiated on observation. Administrative behaviours were agreed by all professionals to dominate the nurses' job and this was substantiated on observation. Educational behaviours featured infrequently, a perception shared by other professionals and confirmed by observation.

How was the role of professional nurses perceived by nurses themselves and by other professionals, many of whom worked closely with them? Did nurses meet their professional, statutory obligations to their patients and to nursing management? Most importantly, what, in essence, as revealed by the findings, is the reality of nurses' job? Did nurses perceive their education, training and professional development as adequate and realistic to help them cope with the nature and demands of their job?

Essentially, nurses perceived their basic role as 'caring' or 'nursing', whereas nurse managers perceived the nurses' role, especially that of ward sister/charge nurse, to be mainly 'managerially' or 'administratively' orientated in terms of its content and functions. However, this point was disputed by the role occupants; many ward sisters (82%) saw their role as a caring one with an added administrative/managerial function. The staff nurses' role was perceived by them to be 'more nursing/teaching' orientated. This paradox in the view of many (90%) nurses and most (72%) doctors produced a dilemma for nurses in their job, which they said affected adversely their motivation and job satisfaction for role requirements for which professionally they said they had 'not been effectively prepared'. They stated the profile, thus described, was 'alien' to their role.

In practice, based on an analysis of the nurses' observed behaviours (Tables 4.3 and 4.4), the findings identified a multidimensional role containing some management components, substantial administration, a nursing element (slightly more for staff nurses than ward sisters/charge nurses), and a minor teaching component (mainly for staff nurses). Many (95%) ward sisters/ charge nurses said they had little if any time for teaching.

During interview, ward sisters on acute medical and surgical wards claimed they spent 10% of their time on direct patient care. On the longstay wards, sisters stated that they spent 50% of their time on direct care. These claims were not borne out during observation. For example, during a 6-hour period in the district health authority (DHA) 1 acute medical ward, the sister averaged 22.96 minutes; in the acute surgical ward, 13.75 minutes; in the longstay ward, 23.83 minutes. Over a 6-hour period in DHA 2, the sister averaged in the acute medical ward 13.75 minutes; in the acute surgical ward, 31.66 minutes; in the longstay ward, 44.58 minutes.

Many nurses, including nurse managers, perceived little difference in practice between the roles of ward sister and staff nurse, as many staff nurses frequently, in the absence of the ward sister, assumed full responsibility for the ward. However, even though this was also the perception of many doctors and officers of the statutory and professional bodies, they additionally said that

Table 4.3 Observations of average time (minutes) spent by six ward sisters/charge nurses on major, predetermined behaviours over a period of six hours in different wards in two district health authorities (DHA)

Behaviour observed	DHA 1			DHA 2		
	Acute medical	Acute surgical	Longstay	Acute medical	Acute surgical	Longstay
1. Managerial	14.28	07.08	12.50	10.83	06.66	16.66
2. Administrative	22.50	24.16	20.16	16.26	12.08	14.66
3. Clinical	22.96	13.75	23.83	13.75	31.66	44.58
Education						
4. Nurses	00.00	00.00	00.00	02.08	00.00	00.00
5. Patients	01.25	00.00	00.00	00.41	01.25	00.00
Communication						
6. Nurses	03.33	07.08	06.66	05.41	08.75	08.75
7. Doctors	12.50	10.83	00.00	07.50	07.08	00.00
8. Patients	04.16	14.16	08.33	05.00	08.33	
						10.00
Time on phone						
9. Giving information	01.25	07.58	09.16	06.65	02.50	00.00
10. Receiving information	07.50	04.16	06.66	04.16	03.75	00.00
11. Direct supervision of nurses	00.00	00.00	00.00	06.25	03.33	00.00
12. Waiting	00.00	00.41	00.00	00.00	00.00	00.00
13. Resting	04.16	05.0	03.75	13.75	06.66	00.00
14. Walking	05.83	07.08	05.00	05.00	06.66	05.75
15. Miscellaneous	00.00	02.08	04.16	02.91	01.25	02.25

staff nurses were more involved in direct nursing care; this was demonstrated clearly in the observed behaviours of staff nurses but not to the extent they perceived. Staff nurses on acute medical and surgical wards during interview said they spent 50% and 55%, repectively, of their time on direct patient care. On observation in DHA 1 acute medical wards, staff nurses spent an average of 33 minutes during a 6-hour period; in acute surgical wards, 21 minutes; in longstay wards, 43.33 minutes. In DHA 2 acute medical wards, they spent 13 minutes; in acute surgical wards 30 minutes; in longstay wards, 43.33 minutes.

Senior nurse managers agreed a 'virtually interchangeable' role for ward sister and staff nurse, with the senior staff nurse assuming full responsibility in the sister's absence, though they perceived the ward sister to have a higher element of managerial behaviour in her job interwoven with administrative behaviour, which they quantified in terms of an 8-hour shift. In this respect, the ward sister's role was perceived to occupy 70% managerial/administrative behaviour; 20% direct patient care; and 10% teaching (nurses and patients). The staff nurses' time during an 8-hour shift was perceived to occupy 30% managerial/administrative behaviour; 45% direct patient care; and 25% teaching.

Many (85%) nurses said that most of the prescribed duties identified in their

THE JOB OF THE NURSE

Table 4.4 Observations of average time (minutes) spent by 16 staff nurses on major, predetermined behaviours over a period of six hours in different wards in two district health authorities (DHA)

Observed behaviour	Acute medical			Acute surgical			Longstay	
	1	2	3	1	2	3	1	2
DHA 1								
1. Managerial	7.91	1.25	11.25	7.08	11.25	15.41	5.00	7.5
2. Administrative	12.91	10.41	15.00	29.16	16.25	24.55	20.83	13.33
3. Clinical	29.58	38.33	33.33	17.91	20.83	12.08	32.08	43.33
Teaching								
4. Nurses	00.00	00.41	00.00	00.00	00.00	00.00	00.00	00.00
5. Patients	00.00	00.00	00.83	00.00	00.00	02.08	06.66	00.00
Communication								
6. Nurses	09.16	07.91	06.66	06.25	13.58	10.41	08.33	00.50
7. Doctors	10.00	04.58	07.91	03.75	07.08	07.50	03.33	05.41
8. Patients	08.33	12.08	07.50	07.50	12.08	05.41	10.00	06.66
Time on phone								
9. Giving information	05.66	00.00	02.90	06.25	01.55	05.00	02.08	01.25
10. Receiving information	01.66	00.41	02.90	00.41	03.33	02.91	00.83	04.58
11. Direct supervision of nurses	2.50	00.00	00.00	07.91	00.00	00.00	00.00	00.00
12. Waiting	00.00	00.00	00.00	00.00	00.00	00.00	00.00	00.00
13. Resting	00.00	06.66	01.25	02.08	00.00	01.25	0.83	00.00
14. Walking	07.91	13.33	02.08	07.91	10.41	08.75	07.91	07.50
15. Miscellaneous	02.50	04.58	03.33	03.75	03.33	04.56	02.08	03.75
DHA 2								
1. Managerial	03.75	01.25	11.25	10.00	02.91	03.33	05.00	05.83
2. Administrative	28.75	20.83	15.41	16.25	17.88	20.83	17.75	09.58
3. Clinical	13.33	17.08	09.88	32.50	25.00	30.00	30.83	43.33
Teaching								
4. Nurses	00.83	31.25	08.33	00.00	00.00	02.50	03.33	00.00
5. Patients	00.00	02.50	00.83	02.08	00.83	00.00	00.00	00.00
Communication								
6. Nurses	07.91	07.50	16.65	07.91	07.50	05.83	07.50	08.75
7. Doctors	12.08	03.33	00.83	07.91	12.08	03.33	04.16	00.00
8. Patients	00.83	00.83	10.41	09.16	02.08	05.41	07.91	17.08
Time on phone								
9. Giving information	10.00	04.16	05.83	03.83	06.25	02.91	02.58	00.00
10. Receiving information	07.91	04.16	00.00	02.50	05.83	04.16	02.19	00.41
11. Direct supervision of nurses	00.00	00.00	00.00	00.00	00.00	05.00	00.93	00.00
12. Waiting	00.00	00.00	00.00	00.00	00.00	00.00	00.00	00.83
13. Resting	00.00	01.66	09.58	00.41	05.41	07.08	00.00	00.00
14. Walking	10.83	04.98	07.08	06.25	10.83	08.33	10.00	09.58
15. Miscellaneous	03.33	00.83	04.16	01.25	03.75	01.25	05.00	04.58

job description were met. Conversely, they were unable to meet fully many of their responsibilities, especially those of caring for their patients and ensuring their safety and wellbeing. Nurses in the main perceived that they had the requisite authority to manage their wards and to care for their patients, despite other evidence in their responses to the contrary.

Most (86%) ward sisters and 95% of staff nurses agreed, to a greater or lesser extent, on their autonomy, insofar as their ability to make what they regarded as key decisions on patient care was fettered most of the time, especially in ensuring the correct resourcing of their wards.

The fact that nurses could not adequately meet many of their responsibilities, compounded by their lack of autonomy, perceived and/or real, are indicators of serious shortcomings of the reality and the proper and professional enactment of their role. In fact the evidence yielded by this study confirms a somewhat disabled role occupant in the sample interviewed and observed. This view is supported by doctors and nurse managers.

The professional development of nurses, perceived by nurses themselves, was inadequate and did not enable their updating in relation to change in general and change in particular relating to their clinical speciality, with which they had to cope. This was exemplified by the fact that approximately 20% of ward sisters interviewed and 43% of staff nurses had not undertaken further training since registration. In this respect 67% of ward sisters and 76% of staff nurses said they could not ensure and improve their professional competence in line with the requirements of the UKCC, even though they wished to do so.

Even though staff nurses were required to adopt 'mentor'/'facilitator' roles and no doubt this function helped some junior nurses, from the evidence given by the staff nurses interviewed most said they lacked support, guidance and counselling, which cast doubt on the practicality and enactment of what they perceived as an additional role.

Many (80%) staff nurses said that the interview during the study was the first time they had been given the opportunity to discuss and examine their role fully. It was clear from the responses that young and relatively inexperienced nurses (1–3 years postregistration) did not receive the encouragement and support that they obviously much craved.

JOB DESCRIPTIONS: A PRESCRIPTION FOR ROLE?

The job descriptions provided (Appendix B) were dated, e.g. some were 10 years old and had not been updated. They were substantial in their identified duties and responsibilities. One senior nurse manager stated that job descriptions were 'historically and traditionally defined, they were developed from the ideas of the Salmon report (1966), and the Mayston report (1969)'. However, nowadays, the manager continued, 'they are changing, broad terms are used, and they are crammed with as much information as possible'.

Newly registered nurses received their job descriptions with their letter of appointment, without discussion and/or explanation. This was subsequently confirmed by a nurse manager. Some newly registered nurses indicated their 'unease' about their being given a role for which they had not been properly prepared, even to the extent of not having the nature and demands of their role explained. The stark implications of these perceived shortcomings are crucial to the nurse, the patient and the organization of health care within these districts, leaving some nurses bewildered about their role. The evidence arising from the study, especially that revealed in subsequent chapters, underline these shortcomings.

The organizational, clinical, technological and educational requirements of the clinical specialities studies make weighty demands on the expertise of professional nurses. Nurses' accountability for their actions in this respect is great, demanding and continuing.

The demands on nurses, especially those of optimally meeting patients' needs, in the perception of nurses themselves and of other professionals, often operate against the heavy odds of uncertainty of staffing levels and workload. The acknowledged multifaceted role of the nurse, including the demanding elements of caring, teaching, administering, managing, communicating, advising and appraising, to mention but a few, mean considerable, regular and frequent adjustment by nurses to the pace, method and technology of their role. However, on observation and discussion, many of these demands were rarely fully met, with nurses stating their concern: 'I seldom have time to communicate with patients because of all the paperwork'. Ward sisters (43%) and staff nurses (54%) said 'It is quicker to use a task approach to care rather than involve the patient, which is too time consuming; you try to ensure the independence of patients, especially their mobility, but it's an uphill struggle because of staff shortages; there is not enough time to supervise learners and auxiliaries who do a lot of the work'. Nurse managers were clearly concerned at some inadequacies of the service that affected the role of the nurse: 'Workload and staffing levels prevent safe standards of practice especially through the lack of supervision of nurses' work' (see Tables 4.3 and 4.4).

In practice much of the direct, 'hands-on' care was given by nursing students (65%) and/or nursing auxiliaries (approximately 66%). This was especially obvious on longstay wards, which were substantially staffed by nursing auxiliaries, many of whom could not be closely supervised because of the shortage of trained and experienced nurses, too many patients, high patient dependency levels and (often) large wards.

How were standards set? Was the care given evaluated? A prerequisite to ensuring proper standard of care is that of evaluating the care given. The responses of ward sisters (34%) and staff nurses (25%) confirmed that the evaluation of patient care did not feature to a great extent in their job. This acknowledgement was substantiated by unit nurse managers (33%) and many doctors (79%). In practice, many nurses said that 'the evaluation of care was done subjectively (visually); defined and agreed criteria were not used regularly'. During periods of observed behaviour (132 hours) there was no evidence of the objective evaluation of patient care. The nursing process was the stated system for the planning and evaluation of patient care in both health districts that was intended to form the framework for individualized patient care. However, many (75%) staff nurses said 'We only use this if it is convenient and proper ward staffing permits'.

The nursing process was frequently alluded to, but wholly in the context of its burden of administration, e.g. patient history taking, care plan formulation and record keeping. Only two ward sisters (10%) and five staff nurses (7%) said they used this system of care regularly. The Merrison report (1979), when referring to standards of care, stated:

> The evidence submitted indicated that the main areas of risk in hospitals related to untrained staff left in charge of wards, inadequate supervision of learners, neglect of basic nursing routines and the employment of agency staff.
>
> *(Para. 13.5, p. 185)*

The report concluded that 'these are serious matters and there is no doubt that nurses are under pressure in many places, and services to patients suffer' (para. 13.6, p. 185). More recently, a report of the Royal College of Nursing (1984) had some difficulty in establishing what was meant by 'standard of care' and stated:

> Standards of care is a difficult concept to discuss simply because there are so many ways to measure standards. But when nurses themselves say that through staff shortages they are no longer able to give a level of care that, as professionals, they know the patient requires, this is a case for real concern.
>
> *(Para. 5, p. 34)*

The evidence gained from the study through interviews and observation of nurses' defined duties indicated marked limitations in nurses addressing 'to a reasonable extent' or 'at all' some of their identified and prescribed duties as listed in their job descriptions. Nurses frequently stated their inability to ensure total patient care, often stating their approach was 'ritualistic and mechanistic in its orientation'.

Twenty-eight responsibilities were studied (see Chapter 5 and Appendix D). All three categories of responsibilities – clinical (7), managerial (12) and education (9) – were perceived by nurses and other professionals only to be met to a limited extent. Key responsibilities, including acknowledging and managing the workload and pressure on colleagues and subordinates, in practice were 'seldom' met.

Most ward sisters in their rating indicated they had little or no control over ensuring the adequacy of resources; many perceived this responsibility being central to the efficiency of their job. Most important, many could not safeguard the wellbeing of patients, ensure high standards of care and give information to patients and relatives, either formally or informally. Many also stated marked limitations to ensuring their own professional competent and development, counselling and teaching of nurses, and effecting the positive health education of their patients. The ratings given by staff nurses to all three categories of their identified responsibilities differed little from those of ward sisters.

Unit nurse managers were divided in their responses on how well nurses met their responsibilities. They emphasized marked limitations to nurses ensuring the adequacy of resources. In practice, they agreed this was their responsibility; nurses could not overturn their decision.

Senior nursing management unequivocally stated their reservations on the feasibility of nurses (ward sisters and staff nurses) being able to fulfil many of their responsibilities clinically, managerially and educationally.

Doctors in the main stated that there were marked limitations to nurses meeting virtually all of the identified responsibilities. Many doctors were unable (because of their stated lack of knowledge) to comment on the educational responsibilities of the professional nurse. Officers of the statutory and professional bodies were somewhat pessimistic as to nurses' ability to meet key clinical responsibilities relating to patient safety and standards of practice. Some managerial and educational responsibilities were also perceived by them to be unsatisfactorily met, prominent among them being: dealing with workload and pressure on colleagues and subordinates, ensuring proper resources, ensuring their personal competence and professional development and effecting the health education of their patients.

PERCEIVED IMPEDIMENTS

Impediments perceived by professionals to nurses' ability to meet their responsibilities included those of unrealistic staffing levels, perceived by them to bear little relationship to the demands of ward organization and administration; reliance on inexperienced, recently registered nurses, inexperienced nursing students and untrained nursing auxiliaries; the burden and excess of paperwork, including much form-filling, report-writing and documentation. On observation of the admission of one patient, a nurse took approximately 45 minutes to complete the voluminous paperwork, most of which was subsequently repeated by a doctor. This was a task that doctors felt could be rationalized to the benefit of nurses, doctors and most importantly the patients. The pace of work was especially emphasized by nurses on surgical wards. The lack of time 'to do things properly', i.e. to supervise staff, talk to patients and their relatives and give direct patient care, was stressful to many nurses; lack of real authority and autonomy was perceived to fetter and limit nurses in making decisions pertinent to their work.

Many (87%) doctors and officers of the nursing statutory and professional bodies perceived the nurses' difficulty in ensuring the confidentiality of patients' information. Doctors said it was impossible for nurses and indeed themselves to ensure the confidentiality of information, because too many professionals had access to patients' notes and 'loose' comments were sometimes made by staff about patients. The extended family, divorced partners and other relatives felt they had a right to patients' information. There was also poor ward design, with lack of ward facilities, including interview rooms and proper screens between beds. The compound effect of these was to enhance the problem of ensuring the confidentiality of patients' information. Adding to this problem, some staff nurses (26%) said that doctors shouted and talked loudly at the foot of the patients' beds; this aggravated the problem by enabling patients in adjacent beds to hear discussions with and/or about individual patients.

The officers of the statutory and professional bodies generally perceived the non-use of the authority and autonomy by some professional nurses, which could be attributed to traditional reasons, i.e. nurses' perceived subordinate role to other professionls, coupled with nurses' lack of assertiveness and their inability to make decisions, as substantially contributing to nurses' inability to meet their statutory obligations. Many nurses were unable to meet responsibilities which they, their managers and the statutory body deemed to be central to the effective, efficient and professional care of their patients, as well as to the wellbeing of their colleagues and nursing students.

From discussion with colleagues and confirmed by officers of the nursing statutory and professional bodies, this situation is not only a 'local' problem, but also prevalent nationally.

Many nurses, including some recently registered nurses, said their initiative and aspirations were often curtailed insofar as they 'did not have a voice' in the running of their wards; paradoxically, frequently, because of staff shortages, in the absence of the ward sister they were obliged to undertake full responsibility for the ward.

Current change in the NHS relating to the training and employment of nurses has introduced another dimension that has affected the aspirations of many nurses. As a preface to Project 2000 the UKCC (1985) agreed a 5-year strategy plan that included among its objectives 'To determine an education and training policy to ensure that nurses, midwives and health visitors who are trained and registered meet the needs of society in the 1990s and beyond.

The needs of society constantly change; therefore, it is realistic to expect nurses to change their attitudes, goals and aspirations. Many newly registered nurses and those wishing to return to work are not able to secure employment. Many are disgruntled and wonder why they bothered to train, but are today's nurses being realistic? Should nurses enter training with a firm belief that on graduation they will automatically be offered a job, and that it will continue for life? No other student entering higher education thinks this way; they know they will not have a guaranteed profession for life, but embark positively on courses that it is hoped will equip them to be well placed to compete for the jobs on offer and they are prepared to relocate.

Nurses must realize and accept that with the enactment of the Community Care Act 1990 (NHS, 1990) and the setting up of hospital trusts (DoH, 1989) there may well be a need for fewer nurses and greater competition for jobs. For example, patients discharged from longstay wards into the community may only need the support of a home help, someone to do their shopping and supportive care from the primary health care service. Is this any different to the care received in a longstay ward? As found in the study, most of the care was carried out by untrained and unqualified staff (65% of nursing students and 66% of nursing auxiliaries) although it could be argued that they were supervised by registered nurses. However, this argument was not upheld by the findings. During interview, ward sisters (90%) and staff nurses (69%) said they monitored the work of nurses, but were unable to give direct supervision, stating 'We have no time to supervise learners and auxiliaries who do a lot of the work'. This view was supported by nurse managers, doctors and officers of the statutory and professional bodies. On observation, little time was spent on the direct supervision of learners or auxiliaries.

Maybe it is time to move away from the concept of nursing as a vocation and in this respect a 'job for life' and move towards a more realistic career structure, with acknowledgement of its inherent advantages and disadvantages. There will always be a need for nurses and change should not undermine the commitment of nurses in the transition from vocation to profession.

DATA DERIVED FROM OBSERVATION OF NURSES' WORK

An essential part of the methodology of the study was the observation of a sample of ward sisters/charge nurses and staff nurses doing their job (Tables 4.3 and 4.4). The sample was randomly selected; six ward sisters (35%, $n=21$) and 16 staff nurses (20%, $n=74$) were observed from the three specialities represented in the study. Each nurse selected was approached and the nature of the observation discussed. The total duration of observation was for ward sisters, 132 hours and for staff nurses, 96 hours. A timetable was constructed and each nurse was observed for three 2-hour periods which sampled their working day, i.e. early morning, mid-morning and afternoon, at 1.5-minute intervals. Nurses were interviewed prior to the first period of observation.

This observation enabled an exploration of 'major' nurses' behaviours (13 said these occurred frequently), and also enabled some comparison to be made of the frequency (as stated by nurses in their interview) and the dominance (identified in job descriptions) of certain behaviours in the nurses' job. The profile of the ward at the time of observation was noted, together with nurses' and the observer's comments.

ANALYSIS

Nurses' behaviours, with few exceptions, were characterized by their frequency, brevity, fragmentation (interrupted by doctors' visit, telephone, etc.) and repetitiveness. They were largely task-based rather than patient-centred.

Throughout periods of nurses' observed behaviours, there was little evidence of sustained interactions with other nurses and patients. Communication within these groups was extremely limited. Also, there was little evidence of any formal education of nurses and patients (health education). Most important, time spent on the supervision of other members of the nursing team was limited. In this respect, nurses in charge often said 'this happens because of personal workload and too much ward administration, and not enough time to teach and/or supervise staff'. The magnitude of the so-called paperwork was exemplified by the provision of patient dependency levels three times a day to nurse managers, together with preparation of the bed state, patient reports, care plans, accident reports, untoward incident reports, requisitioning of resources, admission of patients (often taking up to 45 minutes), transfer and discharge of patients and maintaining links between other departments, including pharmacy, dietetics, outpatients, social work, GP and community nursing service. Of the nurses observed, only two demonstrated managerial behaviours, e.g. deciding, planning, organizing, leading, motivating, monitoring and supervising.

There were only marginal differences in the behaviours observed in clinical specialities and districts. The main differences were that staff nurses engaged more in clinical behaviours than did ward sisters and their managerial behaviours were minimal. Finally, there was an appreciable difference in the extent to which nurses, ward sisters and staff nurses engaged in clinical behaviours on longstay wards.

A statistical analysis of the observation results was carried out, samples of which can be found in Tables 4.5 and 4.6.

Thus observed, the limited time spent by nurses on many of their defined duties and tasks was highlighted. During periods of observation, a record was kept of patients' ward reports and doctors' ward rounds. Ward reports, i.e. the formal reporting to and by the nursing team on patients' care and treatment, and doctors' ward rounds were recorded as separate events. The listed behaviours that were associated with these events (e.g. managerial and administrative), if and when they occurred, were recorded in the appropriate categories in the observation schedule.

The formal reporting by and to nurses on patients' care and treatment was usually brief, lasting about 10 minutes. Five sessions were observed. They

Table 4.5 Analysis of time spent by ward sisters/charge nurses on management and administrative behaviours. Sample, number of 1.5-minute periods spent on behaviour in two hours. Count, number of two-hour periods showing same samples. Percentage, count as % of total time observed

Sample	Count	Cumulative count	Percentage	Cumulative percentage
Management				
2	1	1	5.56	5.56
3	1	2	5.56	11.11
5	2	4	11.11	22.22
6	1	5	5.56	17.78
7	1	6	5.56	33.33
9	1	7	5.56	38.89
10	5	12	27.78	66.67
11	2	14	11.11	77.78
12	3	17	16.67	94.44
13	1	18	5.56	100.00
Administration				
8	2	2	11.11	11.11
9	1	3	5.56	16.67
10	2	5	11.11	27.78
11	2	7	11.11	38.89
13	2	9	11.11	50.00
14	2	11	11.11	61.11
15	2	13	11.11	72.22
16	1	14	5.56	77.78
18	1	15	5.56	83.33
22	2	17	11.11	94.44
23	1	18	5.56	100.00

Table 4.6 Analysis of time spent by staff nurses on communication with patients (formal and informal). Sample, number of 1.5-minute periods spent on behaviour in two hours. Count, number of two-hour periods showing same samples. Percentage, count as % of total time observed

Sample	Count	Cumulative count	Percentage	Cumulative percentage
0	6	6	12.50	12.50
1	2	8	4.17	16.67
2	2	10	4.17	20.83
3	1	11	2.08	22.92
4	8	19	16.67	39.58
5	5	24	10.42	50.00
6	3	27	6.25	56.25
7	5	32	10.42	66.67
8	2	34	4.17	70.83
9	4	38	8.33	79.17
11	3	41	6.25	85.42
12	3	44	6.25	91.67
13	2	46	4.17	95.83
14	1	47	2.08	97.92
16	1	48	2.08	100.00

essentially consisted of the nurse in charge informing the ward team of special tasks and procedures to be undertaken. There was little dialogue, but much note taking. There was no in-depth discussion or evaluation of patient care. These sessions were hurried and nurses claimed that was due to workload. When nurses were questioned as to the value of these sessions they said 'They tend to be too hurried and allow little time for proper discussion'.

There were many (10) 'mini', usually conducted by house officers and registrars, and two 'major' ward rounds observed. The latter were detailed and lengthy, some alleged by nurses to last 3 4 hours. They showed little real involvement of the nurse in charge, whose role centred mainly on associated clerical duties, i.e. ensuring that all medical reports, charts, X-rays, etc. were available and up-to-date. In the context of the findings it is interesting to note that some two decades ago, the Briggs report (1972), citing the evidence of a work study (source not identified) on ward sisters' activities, stated:

> the vast majority of ward sisters' activities may each last for less than one minute; the pattern is one of frequent interruption and multiple responsibilities, often for minute details. We regard it as imperative to find some ways of relieving the burdens of ward sisters, and freeing them from day-to-day minutiae so that they can devote their attention to the overall planning of care in their ward, with more time to exercise their clinical and teaching skills.
>
> *(Para. 128, p. 42)*

Even though some wards employ part-time (mornings only) ward clerks, ward sisters and staff nurses said this made 'some difference' insofar as it 'freed' them to undertake what they regarded to be their job, the direct care of their patients. Understandably, in the light of the often expressed and observed inordinate workload and perceived understaffing of many wards, little time was recorded during periods of observation of ward sisters and staff nurses 'waiting' and 'resting' between activities, even the taking of approved 'rest' periods.

The observed behaviours of nurses demonstrated their variety, brevity and fragmentation (behaviours which readily and consistently alternated) and created in their wake, stress for the role occupant. Nurses were required frequently to change pace and direction while simultaneously attempting to provide a service of care.

Generally the findings showed considerable differences between nurses' stated behaviours of their role during interview, their prescribed behaviours identified in their job descriptions and the observed behaviours. For example, ward sisters in both districts during interview stated that managerial and clinical behaviours were dominant in their role. However, on observation they demonstrated few managerial behaviours, e.g. planning, monitoring, leading, supervising and motivating. Also, despite statements to the contrary, they spent very little time on direct patient care.

Staff nurses' perceived and prescribed behaviours on observation showed differences in their frequency, especially for managerial and administrative behaviours and education of nurses and health education of patients (for details see Tables 4.3 and 4.4, Appendix C).

The role of the nurse is a complex issue, especially in an ever changing society and National Health Service. It is the subject of much research and discussion, including the publications already listed under 'Role' in Chapter 3, as well as the following: Katz and Kahn (1966), Pembrey (1980), Aiken (1981), Hingley et al. (1984), Hingley and Cooper (1986), Martinko and Gardner (1985), RCN (1988), UKCC (1989, 1992) and Seccombe and Ball (1992).

This chapter has looked at the nurses' role in general terms. The following chapters will examine and discuss elements of the nurses' role, starting with nurses' accountability.

The framework for the structured interviews was substantially based on nurses' job descriptions and on information obtained during pre-pilot and pilot studies.

Nurses' accountability and its role-related elements | 5

BACKGROUND

The responsibilities of the professional nurse are many and onerous. Nurses are legally accountable for their responsibilities, which are specified in their job description and which are underlined and amplified in the *Code of Professional Conduct for Nurses, Midwives and Health Visitors* (UKCC, 1984, 1992).

This chapter examines nurses' responsibilities in the context of the role of the professional nurse in the hospital environment. Before the examination of nurses' responsibilities and the perceptions of professionals on the ability of nurses to meet the responsibilities for which they are accountable, a discussion of the legal and professional framework within which nurses practise may help to underline the reality of the demands of this aspect of the nurses' role.

Nurses' accountability and responsibility are influenced by the extent of their authority (power to make decisions) and their autonomy (freedom to make decisions) in relation to their responsibilities for which they are accountable by virtue of their status as registered nurses. In this respect Rowbottom and Billis (1987) referred to 'the impossibility of simple and blanket answers to the question of how much autonomy a professional should be allowed' and to the fact that 'in large organizations many problems stem from unclear responsibility' (paras 2/1, pp. 126/7).

A recent report of the Audit Commission (1991) exposed one of the grey areas relating to nurses' responsibility:

> At present on many wards there is a lack of clear responsibility for making decisions affecting the care given to a patient. Staff nurses and the ward sister are accountable, but neither feels fully responsible. The nurse caring for the patient may be required to refer significant decisions to the nurse in charge who is less likely to know the full picture.
>
> *(Para. (i), p. 24)*

These views were certainly evident in the study. Many nurses said they had the responsibility to care for patients but in reality they were not empowered or free to make decisions that ensured that these responsibilities were properly met. Is this really a satisfactory answer? Nurses must realize that the responsibility to care for their patients is entirely their remit. They fail to understand that it is not sufficient to say 'we request help but are often refused'. It is unequivocally their responsibility to ensure that the requested help is given, if in their professional opinion the situation would otherwise result in not being able to ensure the care, safety and wellbeing of their patients.

The profession must endeavour to define and clarify precisely the role of the nurse in respect of their responsibility for which they are legally accountable. Increased responsibility brings with it increased accountability. Responsibility and accountability have clear implications for nurses and their patients insofar as nurses are answerable for their working decisions to their employer, their statutory body (the UKCC), the patient and society.

Batey and Lewis (1982) perceived responsibility as 'A charge for which one in answerable. The focus is on the charge, not on how or to whom the answering should or would occur'. The authors perceive accountability as 'The fulfilment of a formal obligation to disclose to referent others the purposes, principles, procedures, relationships, results, income and expenditures for which one has authority' (paras. 1/3, pp. 10/15).

One of the problems nurses face is knowing to whom they are accountable, i.e. the unit nurse manager, senior nurse manager, or general manager? In the study, some staff nurses in their responses were obviously unclear. Some had difficulty accepting their accountability to their own statutory body. Many felt that because they perceived they could not remedy a problem then they could not be held responsible or accountable. The situation was further aggravated by senior managers who believed that their own position in the context of their authority was greatly diminished, resulting in 'often having little control over decisions which affect nurses'.

This situation is not at all surprising in light of events relating to professional officers' accountability in the wake of the Griffiths report (1983). At the time, the President of the RCN made the point that the report threatened to deprive nurses of the right to manage patient services (RCN, 1983). This view was not in isolation, but one of many comments which questioned the validity of the report, e.g. Evans and Maxwell (1984) and Davidmann (1984).

Was this pessimistic view of 'a threat to nurses' justified? There is nothing in the Griffiths report that said that nurses could not apply for (in fact it encouraged nurses to apply for) senior jobs in the management of patient services. In an interview with the *Daily Telegraph*, November 1983, Roy Griffiths made the following point: 'The General Manager is going to be the person best suited to the job, regardless of profession and it can quite easily be a nurse'.

However, the profession was concerned, because they envisaged that not many nurses would be appointed as General Managers and a situation would arise as described in the DHSS (1984) health circular which stated 'On matters relating to the fulfilment of the general managers' responsibility professional chief officers will be accountable to the general manager for the day to day performance of their management functions' (para. 7, p. iii). Nurses were worried that they would be accountable to someone other than a nurse. Some of these fears were realized with the removal from post of some chief nursing officers following the appointment of general managers.

During recent discussion (1993) with some chief professional officers, it was stated by them that their position continues to remain unclear and devoid of any real authority. The profession needs to take cognizance of these dilemmas and ensure that senior and chief professional officers are given the opportunity to gain the necessary skills required for the post of general manager, and these should be embodied in training from studentship throughout their career as an important part of their professional development.

THE LEGAL AND PROFESSIONAL FRAMEWORK

Nurses' accountability is central to the integrity of the role of the professional nurse. In a legal sense accountability may involve liability. Nurses are accountable for their practice. The Code of Professional Conduct (UKCC, 1984, 1992) together with the subsequent amendments (UKCC, 1987, 1989) amplify and clarify this accountability.

The Nurses, Midwives and Health Visitors Act 1979, together with the EEC nursing and midwifery directives (EEC, 1977, 1989), underline directly or indirectly the activities of nurses responsible for general care, including the co-ordination of provision laid down by law in respect of activities of nurses responsible for general care.

In meeting their many demanding and varied responsibilities, nurses are obliged by statute to uphold the standards of practice that are embodied in the *Code of Professional Conduct* (UKCC, 1992) and which are further clarified and amplified in the documents *Exercising Accountability* (UKCC, 1989) and *The Scope of Professional Practice* (UKCC, 1992). The use of the words 'accountable' and 'accountability' provide the central focus 'for the expectation that practitioners will conduct themselves in the manner the *Code of Professional Conduct* describes' (UKCC, 1989, para. 2, p. 6). In reality, if nurses fail to uphold the standards of practice thus defined, the ultimate penalty that can be exacted by the nursing statutory body for proven non-compliance by 'action or omission' (UKCC, 1984, para. 2, p. 2) that takes place 'in their professional practice where they are obliged to make judgments, in a wide variety of circumstances, whether engaged in current practice or not, and whether on or off duty' (UKCC, 1989, para. 3, p. 6) is that she, for 'misconduct or otherwise, may be removed from the register of qualified nurses' (*Nurses, Midwives and Health Visitors Act 1979*, para. 12(1)).

Pyne (1985) summarized the code of conduct in general, and nurses' accountability in particular, in the following way:

> The role of the practitioner is to serve the public interest and that of patients; never, by action or omission place a patient's condition or safety at risk; draw attention to those places where safe standards of practice are endangered or impossible; care for and about colleagues, in respect both of their development and workload; and take every opportunity to sustain and improve their knowledge and professional competence.

EXERCISING ACCOUNTABILITY

In light of the foregoing demands, are nurses enabled or disabled to a greater or lesser extent, by the environment in which they work as well as by the elements of their role? And, in this context, do a lack of resources, human and material, together with a limited degree of authority and autonomy to make decisions appropriate to their role and status and especially to the professional care of their patients, disable them in their endeavour to meet these obligations? (The findings of this study show substantial evidence to the contrary.) Do the authority and autonomy of the nurses' role enable them to fulfil their constant and demanding responsibilities? Many nurses, though acknowledging their authority, said they lacked the necessary autonomy. (This will be discussed in Chapter 6.) What happens should nurses fail to meet these responsibilities, for whatever reason?

The preface to the *Code of Professional Conduct* (UKCC, 1992) is both comprehensive and explicit in its demands for nurses' accountability in the fulfilment of their responsibilities as practitioners on the UKCC's register and, in this respect, states:

> Each registered nurse, midwife and health visitor shall act, at all times, in such a manner as to justify public trust and confidence, to uphold and enhance the good standing and reputation of the profession, to serve the interests of society and above all to safeguard the interests of patients and clients.
>
> *(Para. 1)*

The code continues: 'Each registered nurse, midwife and health visitor is accountable for his or her practice' (para. 2).

These legal requirements effectively summarize and embody the central and binding demands on nurses in the execution of their onerous responsibilities in the context of an often blurred role and its perceived, if not actual, limited authority and autonomy. The way nurses perceived they performed their role, i.e. met their responsibility and accountability by properly carrying out their many duties and tasks for which they are responsible and met their associated accountability to their employer, the UKCC and their patients, was established through in-depth interviews lasting on average one hour. The interviews were conducted with ward sisters ($n = 21$), staff nurses ($n = 74$), nurse managers ($n = 8$), doctors ($n = 29$) and representative officers of the nursing statutory and professional bodies ($n = 3$). The interviews focused on nurses' defined responsibilities, i.e. responsibilities defined in their job descriptions and outlined in the code of conduct.

The principal objectives for studying nurses' responsibilities were to assess the reality of nurses' accountability, to establish how completely nurses themselves and other professionals perceived that nurses met their responsibilities and to identify any impediments to these being met.

A five-point scale was used to determine how far it was possible for nurses to meet their responsibilities. The following rating was used:

Completely:	Always
To a reasonable degree:	Most times
On the whole, Yes:	It depends, sometimes
Not usually:	Seldom, if at all
Impossible:	Never

Each responsibility was rated on a range varying from 'Completely' to 'Impossible'. Three categories including 28 responsibilities were studied: clinical (7), managerial (12) and educational (9). Tables 5.1 and 5.2 give the nurses' responses. For information on how other professionals responded, see Appendix D.

COMMENT

It is evident from Tables 5.1 and 5.2 that many ward sisters and staff nurses found it impossible to meet 'Completely' many of their responsibilities. The impediments perceived by them, some of which have already been discussed in previous chapters, can be summarized as those relating to a lack of manpower, high patient dependency, and a heavy burden of ward administration. They often stated that they could not always ensure safe standards of practice because of workload and staffing levels. Nurse managers generally agreed with these views, acknowledging nurses' inability to meet key responsibilities. One stated: 'The pressures on ward staff are tremendous; it is difficult for them to deliver the goods'.

Doctors in the main voiced more forcefully the nurses' inability to cope with the pressures and workload of the job: 'Nurses can do little about the workload, they can request help but often do not get it'. 'If help isn't available,

Table 5.1 Rating by ward sisters/charge nurses ($n=21$) of their ability to meet their prescribed responsibilities

Responsibility	Com-pletely	To a reason-able degree	On the whole, Yes	Not usually	Impos-sible
Clinical					
1. Act always to promote and safeguard the wellbeing of patients	33.33	38.10	28.57	–	–
2. Take account of the customs of patients	42.56	42.86	14.29	–	–
3. Carry out medical instructions	52.38	33.33	14.29	–	–
4. Ensure high standards of care	42.86	42.86	14.29	–	–
5. Respect the confidential information of patients	95.24	4.76	–	–	–
6. Ensure safe standards of practice (supervision of work)	47.62	28.57	19.05	–	4.76
7. Inform persons as appropriate of patients' progress (relatives, doctor, senior nursing manager)	57.14	19.05	19.05	4.76	–
Managerial					
1. Work in a collaborative manner with other healthcare professionals	61.90	38.10	–	–	–
2. Make known to an appropriate person/authority any conscientious objection relative to professional practice	95.24	4.76	–	–	–
3. Ensure the adequacy of resources	–	19.05	38.10	33.33	9.52
4. Make known to an appropriate person/authority circumstances which militate against safe standards of practice	85.71	14.29	–	–	–
5. Have regard to the workload on colleagues	19.05	9.52	42.86	23.81	4.76
6. Have regard to the workload on subordinates	19.05	9.52	42.86	23.81	4.76
7. Have regard to the pressures on colleagues	19.05	9.52	42.86	23.81	4.76
8. Have regard to the pressures on subordinates	19.05	9.52	38.10	28.57	4.76
9. Take action to reduce the workload on colleagues	–	–	38.10	38.10	23.81
10. Take action to reduce the workload on subordinates	–	–	38.10	38.10	23.81
11. Take action to reduce undue pressures on colleagues	–	–	42.86	38.10	19.05
12. Take action to reduce the pressures on subordinates	–	–	42.86	38.10	19.05

Table 5.1—*continued*

Responsibility	Com-pletely	To a reason-able degree	On the whole, Yes	Not usually	Impos-sible
Educational					
1. Improve own professional competence – skills and knowledge (specific)	33.33	47.62	14.29	4.76	–
2. Assist colleagues to develop professional competence (skills and knowledge)	28.57	52.38	14.29	4.76	–
3. Assist subordinates to develop professional competence (passing on of skills and knowledge)	47.62	42.86	9.52	–	–
4. Teach subordinates	57.14	23.81	14.29	4.76	–
5. Advise patients (health education)	52.38	19.05	9.52	14.29	4.76
6. Counsel staff as appropriate	47.62	28.57	23.81	–	–
7. Ensure own professional development (general)	33.33	42.86	14.29	4.76	4.76
8. Prepare programmes of training (nursing techniques and ward management)	42.86	19.05	23.81	14.29	–
9. Act as assessor (ward-based examinations)	95.24	–	–	4.76	–

they do the job, usually'. During observation, even though the workload was heavy, nurses could have organized their time and planning of tasks more effectively. This is one aspect of nurses' training that requires more thought and development and is discussed further in Chapter 9.

The officers of the nursing statutory and professional bodies acknowledged in general terms the nurses' difficulty in meeting their obligations, identifying impediments including 'Nurses have never been good in taking decisions; this is part of nurses' non-assertiveness' and 'they are totally intimidated by doctors and managers'. Many nurses interviewed stated their difficulty and the associated dilemma for them regarding their commitment to the patient and their loyalty to nurse management. In this context some nurses found difficulty 'informing their statutory body on certain shortcomings in the ward environment, which prevented them meeting their responsibilities following unheeded requests to management'.

In the situation depicted, nurses are obliged to ensure the proper resourcing of their wards and 'report to an appropriate person or authority any circumstances in which safe and appropriate care for patients cannot be provided' (UKCC, 1992, para. 3). The present professional and legal

Table 5.2 Rating by staff nurses ($n = 74$) of their ability to meet their prescribed responsibilities

Responsibility	Com-pletely	To a reason-able degree	On the whole, Yes	Not usually	Impos-sible
Clinical					
1. Act always to promote and safeguard the wellbeing of patients	50.54	47.30	12.16	–	–
2. Take account of the customs of patients	17.57	63.51	18.92	–	–
3. Carry out medical instructions	70.27	24.32	5.41	–	–
4. Ensure high standards of care	31.08	62.16	6.76	–	–
5. Respect the confidential information of patients	90.54	8.11	1.35	–	–
6. Ensure safe standards of practice (supervision of work)	48.65	40.54	10.81	–	–
7. Inform persons as appropriate of patients' progress (relatives, doctor, senior nursing manager)	83.78	6.76	4.05	5.41	–
Managerial					
1. Work in a collaborative manner with other healthcare professionals	1.35	27.03	22.47	21.62	27.03
2. Make known to an appropriate person/authority any conscientious objection relative to professional practice	41.89	24.32	22.97	8.11	2.70
3. Ensure the adequacy of resources	6.76	24.32	44.59	14.86	9.46
4. Make known to an appropriate person/authority circumstances which militate against safe standards of practice	5.41	24.32	45.95	14.86	9.46
5. Have regard to the workload on colleagues	5.41	24.32	45.95	14.86	9.46
6. Have regard to the workload on subordinates	5.41	22.97	47.30	14.86	9.46
7. Have regard to the pressures on colleagues	–	6.76	21.62	39.19	32.43
8. Have regard to the pressures on subordinates	–	6.71	21.62	39.19	32.43
9. Take action to reduce the workload on colleagues	–	5.41	22.97	39.19	32.43
10. Take action to reduce the workload on subordinates	–	6.76	21.62	39.19	32.43
11. Take action to reduce undue pressures on colleagues	18.92	58.11	20.27	2.70	–
12. Take action to reduce the pressures on subordinates	8.11	60.81	21.62	6.76	2.70

Table 5.2—*continued*

Responsibility	Com-pletely	To a reason-able degree	On the whole, Yes	Not usually	Impos-sible
Educational					
1. Improve own professional competence – skills and knowledge (specific)	24.32	62.16	13.51	–	–
2. Assist colleagues to develop professional competence (skills and knowledge)	32.43	47.30	13.51	6.76	–
3. Assist subordinates to develop professional competence (passing on of skills and knowledge)	54.05	29.73	10.81	2.70	2.70
4. Teach subordinates	17.57	39.19	14.86	28.38	–
5. Advise patients (health education)	22.97	45.95	24.32	4.05	2.70
6. Counsel staff as appropriate	17.57	32.43	12.16	36.49	1.35
7. Ensure own professional development (general)	91.78	1.37	–	4.11	2.74
8. Prepare programmes of training (nursing techniques and ward management)	75.68	17.57	6.76	–	–
9. Act as assessor (ward-based examinations)	9.45	–	–	–	90.54

requirement in the *Code of Professional Conduct* (UKCC, 1992) and the *Nurses, Midwives and Health Visitors Act* 1979 demands that nurses can be called to account for alleged breaches and, if these are proven, they face the ultimate sanction of their name being removed from the Register. This is just and proper in the interest of patient care and safety. Nurses must always ensure that their statutory obligations are understood fully and are met, despite any inadequacies and/or impediments of the organization in which they work.

They must realize that the legislation is not at fault, but the system in which it operates is flawed. Nurses feel uneasy about challenging the system for fear of loss of job; they anticipate reprisals and strictures on career progression. Whether these expressed fears are valid or not, they may prevent nurses from reporting identified inadequacies in the system. However, nurses must realize that these fears, real or imagined, are not a justifiable excuse in law and they must use the authority of their position as a registered nurse to protect themselves and resolve perceived problems as advised by the UKCC: 'nurses must seek remedies – rather than silently tolerate poor standards' (para. 4, p.

7). If nurses do nothing they are as guilty as those who allow the situation to arise and continue without remedy.

This situation is recognized by the statutory body (UKCC, 1989), which acknowledges tensions in the clinical environment: 'In many clinical situations there may be a tension between the maintenance of standards and the availability and use of resources, e.g. where patients or clients seem likely to be placed in jeopardy and/or inadequacy of resources; and, where valuable resources are being used inappropriately' (para. 4, p. 7).

In the light of these anomalies and shortcomings of the role, what tensions are created? The UKCC (1989) underlines: 'Failure to make concerns known renders practitioners vulnerable to complaint to their regulatory body for failing to satisfy its standards and places their registration status in jeopardy' (para. 1, p. 8). Despite the foregoing statement, the UKCC (1989) recognizes: 'In many clinical situations there may be a tension between the maintenance of standards and the availability and use of resources, e.g. where patients or clients seem likely to be placed in jeopardy and/or standards of practice endangered; where the staff in such settings are at risk because of the pressure of work and/or inadequacy of resources; and, where valuable resources are being used inappropriately' (para. 4, p. 7). Explicit in the *Nurses, Midwives and Health Visitors Act 1979* is the responsibility of nurses for the delivery, standard and quality of patient care. Implicit in this requirement of quality is nurses' responsibility for promoting and safeguarding the physical, mental and social well-being of patients, coupled with nurses' responsibility for their own professional development, including the skills, knowledge and expertise to enable them to meet continuing and increasing job demands. Nurses are accountable for their practice and, in this respect, must continually refresh and update their knowledge and skills, to sustain and improve their professional competence.

SUMMARY

The UKCC (1989), when discussing accountability, acknowledged 'the primacy of the interests of the public and the patient whose interests must predominate over those of practitioner and profession', and 'the exercise by each practitioner of personal professional accountability in such a manner as to respect the primacy of those interests' (para. 3, p. 6). It is evident from discussions with nurses and other professionals that this primacy of interests is difficult to sustain. Many nurses have difficulty meeting, either wholly or in part, many of their prescribed responsibilities to their professional satisfaction.

The concerns voiced by nurses, which were often agreed to by other professionals, unveiled a situation that requires urgent resolution in the interests of professional integrity in facilitating quality patient care. There is clear evidence from these findings that many nurses cannot always ensure the safety of their patients. They do not have sufficient time, because of other duties, to talk to their patients and discuss with them their care, progress and health education. In addition, nurses acknowledged difficulty in ensuring the independence of their patients and including them in their care programme, stating 'You try to ensure the independence of patients but it's an uphill struggle largely because of a lack of resources. For example, to get patients mobile often requires two nurses; if we haven't got them we cannot do it'.

Ward sisters (95%) and staff nurses (90%) expressed difficulty and frustration, due to the overwhelming burden of administration, in not being able to involve themselves in the direct care of their patients and in the proper education and supervision of untrained and unqualified staff. A ward sister stated: 'It is difficult to safeguard patients and ensure safe standards of practice as there is not enough time to supervise learners and auxiliaries who do a lot of the work'. Many staff were concerned that because of staff shortages, they had difficulty minimizing workload and pressure on colleagues and junior staff. For example, of the ward sisters ($n = 21$) interviewed, none were able 'completely' or even 'to a reasonable degree' to take action to reduce the workload on colleagues or subordinates. Many (71%) had difficulty acknowledging and reducing pressures on colleagues and subordinates.

Staff nurses experienced the same difficulties (Table 5.2). These inadequacies were known to nurse managers who from discussion showed concern but acknowledged 'We only have reduced resources which are clearly inadequate, much of the time'. The situation was summarized by officers of the statutory and professional bodies: 'Ensuring high standards of nursing care presents a very unequal picture nationally. Many constraints hinder nurses ensuring the patients' wellbeing, high standards of care and safe standards of practice, including staffing levels and workload'.

Generally, nurses' statements about behaviours in relation to their accountability and the exercising of their responsibilities were closely related to those observed, e.g. they had little say in the resourcing of their wards, ensuring of safe standards of practice, supervision of staff, teaching and education of staff and patients, involvement in direct patient care or communication with patients, and in ensuring or enabling their professional development.

Much has been written and stated about nurses' accountability and responsibility (Salmon, 1966; Hall, 1968; Mayeroff, 1971; Briggs, 1972; Hardy and Conway, 1978; Merrison, 1979; Batey and Lewis, 1982; Lanara, 1982; RCN, 1982, 1983, 1988; DoH Nursing Division, 1989; UKCC, 1989, 1992; Audit Commission, 1991, 1992; Seccombe and Ball, 1992). In the following chapter the nurses' authority and autonomy will be examined and discussed together with the relationship between these and the exercising of nurses' accountability.

6 | Nurses' authority and autonomy in the context of their responsibility and accountability

The UKCC (1989) gives clear, comprehensive information to nurses on responsibilities for which they are accountable:

> While accepting their responsibilities and doing their best to fulfil them, practitioners on its register will ensure that the reality of their clinical environment and practice is made known to and understood by appropriate persons or authorities, doing this as an expression of their personal, professional accountability exercised in the public interest. An essential part of this process is the making of contemporaneous and accurate records of the consequences for patients and clients if they have not been given the care they require . . . No practitioner will find support in the Code or from the UKCC for the contention that genuinely held concerns should not be expressed or, if expressed, should attract censure.
>
> *(Para. 3, p. 9)*

These statements are unequivocal. However, even though the statutory body is well aware of the environment in which nurses strive to meet their responsibilities, the UKCC does not give any direction on the many problems which confront nurses, often fettering them in ensuring their accountability. This is particularly evident in the lack of clarification and/or guidelines on nurses' authority and autonomy, matters frequently addressed over the decades by the professional body (RCN, 1982, 1983, 1988).

Responsibility, authority, autonomy and accountability are viewed by some authors as being inextricably linked (Batey and Lewis, 1982). The authors perceive 'responsibility and authority as necessary conditions for both autonomy and accountability'. They suggest, 'It is illogical and inappropriate for an organisation to hold a department or an individual accountable for those activities over which the department or individual has no authority' (para. 6, p. 13).

Confusion arises when nurses' accountability is limited because they can claim only authority of expert knowledge but not of their position as professional practitioners. This clearly is untenable for the nurse in charge, who is frequently called upon to make decisions on the care of their patients, but does not have the power to ensure the resources required to deliver that care. However, nurses must understand that autonomy does not mean total freedom to do as one chooses, as explained by Mayeroff (1971): 'Autonomy means dependence on others, . . . it assumes self-understanding; without such understanding I get in my own way and go round in circles' (paras 1/2, pp. 57/59).

CONCEPTS AND PERSPECTIVES

Nurses must have confidence in themselves and in their superiors' acknowledgement in their authority and freedom to make legitimate decisions about the care and management of their patients, and the inevitable related resources. Authority is described by Batey and Lewis (1982), as: 'the rightful (legitimate) power to fulfil a charge' (para. 5, p. 14).

Authority to act is delegated. It is inevitably and, in my view, intrinsically related to the integrity of the operation of the role of the professional nurse. In its absence, the nurses' role is reduced to one that is passive and non-influential.

The sphere of authority of the ward sister was stated by the Salmon report (1966), to be: 'readily recognised since one ward is physically separate from another' (para. 4.13, p. 32). The report also stated: 'The tradition in general nursing has been that a Ward Sister is considered to be in control of her ward, whether or not she is temporarily absent' (para. 4.14, p. 32), and the report linked the 'satisfaction' of ward sisters with their job to the fact that each exercised decentralized control and substantially delegated authority. 'Apart from their authority (structural) over their own staff, their personal (sapiential) authority (the right, vested in a person, to be heard by reason of expertness or knowledge), is recognised by all with whom they have dealings' (para. 4.15, p. 32).

The Salmon Committee, in attempting to rationalize the nurses' job, in the view of many experienced nurses, also undermined the ward sisters' authority. This point was voiced at an RCN seminar (1982): 'Concern was expressed over the extent to which the ward sister's role had been eroded and recommended that the full responsibility should be restored. Accountability should be matched by the necessary authority to control the environment of care' (para. 4, p. 2).

During interviews there was evidence of nurses' lack of authority, which was especially noted during periods of observed behaviour where, for example, the nurse in charge could not secure the proper staffing of a busy surgical ward, nor control the activities within the ward. For example, when nine patients, prepared for theatre, had to be escorted to and from theatre by a trained nurse (hospital's policy), repeated requests for staff went unacknowledged, even to the extent that the staff nurse was refused extra cover to enable an official meal break. Ward sisters (60%) and staff nurses (75%) stated: 'We have no control over the nature or the number of staff on a ward, especially agency nurses'. 'We can inform the nurse manager about patient dependency levels but we cannot ensure staffing levels to ensure patients' needs are met'. A staff nurse said 'When sister is in charge and needs extra staff, she can get them; when I am in charge and request extra staff, it is refused; a unit manager has even told me that coping without, will help me show them I am capable of running a ward, if I want to secure a ward sister post'.

In contrast, some nurse managers presented a different perspective. 'Managers say "yes", staff have the requisite authority and autonomy; staff say "no". Nurses are given as much rope as they can safely manage'. One senior manager commented, 'Nurses' authority comes down to having confidence in staff; it depends on the boss'. On the evidence of the study, nurses were not clear as to their role authority and autonomy, e.g. when nurses were asked about the presence of these elements in their role, the majority agreed they had the requisite authority to make decisions but had little or no autonomy to act on those decisions (Tables 6.1 and 6.2).

However, as can be seen from the responses in Chapter 5, Table 5.1, it is clear that many do not have the authority to enable them to meet their responsibilities. Doctors were decisive in their responses about the absence and/or limitation of nurses' power and freedom to make decisions on the care of their patients and the management of their ward, which they attributed to 'being frightened of their superiors to act', and 'doctors and nurse managers prevent nurses doing their job; nurses do not have the power to challenge their decisions and practices'.

The statutory and professional bodies rationalized the foregoing situation, stating 'Nurses have authority but fail to use it because of their lack of assertiveness and for traditional reasons many feel subordinate to doctors and other professionals, especially some senior doctors who intimidate them'. Despite these somewhat contradictory views, virtually all professionals taking part in the study acknowledged the 'relevance and importance' of nurses' power and freedom to make decisions enabling the care of the patient and their own confidence and job satisfaction. The reasons for exploring nurses' authority and autonomy were to establish the presence and reality of these elements in their role.

A three-point scale was used to assess authority:

Yes: Nurses perceived the requisite authority
No: Nurses perceived absence of authority
Not sure: Nurses uncertain as to extent of authority

A four-point scale was used to assess autonomy:

Extremely free: Nurses' wide-ranging freedom, most of the time
Very free: Some limitations, no major constraints
Free: It depends on the situations, some constraints
Not very free: Limited freedom, many constraints

For details of the responses of nurses and other professionals, see Tables 6.1, 6.2 and 6.3.

Table 6.1 Rating by nurses and other professionals or nurses' authority to manage wards, in district health authorities 1 and 2

Grade/profession	Acute medical (n=48)			Acute surgical (n=65)			Longstay (n=17)			n
	Yes	No	Not sure	Yes	No	Not sure	Yes	No	Not sure	
Ward sister/charge nurse	5	1	–	6	4	1	3	1	–	21
Staff nurse	23	8	1	30	3	4	4	1	–	74
Unit nurse manager	2	–	–	2	–	–	2	–	–	6
Doctor	3	3	2	7	8	–	2	3	1	29
Total number of responses	33	12	3	45	15	5	11	5	1	130
Percentage of speciality responses	69	25	6	69	23	8	65	29	6	

COMMENT

For convenience and to enable a comparison of the responses of professionals, the combined results of both health authorities are given under each clinical speciality.

On acute medical wards the majority of ward sisters (5, 83%) perceived they had the requisite authority to manage their wards and care for their patients. Among staff nurses, this authority for the two functions was perceived by 23 (72%) and 24 (74%), respectively. Unit nurse managers concurred with this

Table 6.2 Rating by nurses and other professionals of nurses' authority to care for their patients, in district health authorities 1 and 2

Grade/profession	Acute medical (n = 48)			Acute surgical (n = 65)			Longstay (n = 17)			n
	Yes	No	Not sure	Yes	No	Not sure	Yes	No	Not sure	
Ward sister/charge nurse	5	1	–	6	4	1	3	1	–	21
Staff nurse	24	8	–	31	3	3	4	1	–	74
Unit nurse manager	2	–	–	2	–	–	2	–	–	6
Doctor	3	3	2	7	8	–	2	4	–	29
Total number of responses	34	12	2	46	15	4	11	6	–	130
Percentage of speciality responses	71	25	4	71	23	6	65	35	–	

perception, though the majority of doctors (5, 63%), disagreed and/or were not sure.

In relation to autonomy many ward sisters (4, 66%) perceived considerable constraints on their freedom to make decisions, some (2, 33%) acknowledging the requisite autonomy. The majority of staff nurses (31, 97%) perceived marked constraints on their freedom to operate effectively as registered nurses, especially when in charge of the ward. The two unit managers were divided in their responses, one acknowledged marked limitations to nurses' freedom and one acknowledging some limitations. Doctors (8, 100%) without exception perceived marked constraints.

On acute surgical wards, sisters were divided on the question of their authority; 6 (55%) agreed and 5 (45%) disagreed. The majority of staff nurses (30, 81% and 31, 84%, respectively) perceived the requisite authority to manage their wards (when in charge) and care for their patients. unit nurse managers (2, 100%) perceived nurses had the requisite authority. However, many doctors (8, 53%) disagreed with this perception.

In relation to nurses' autonomy the majority of ward sisters (10, 90%) and most staff nurses (34, 91%) perceived marked constraints on their freedom to act. Unit nurse managers (2, 100%) acknowledged some, though in their view not disabling, limitations to nurses' freedom. Doctors (15, 100%) perceived some constraints on nurses' freedom, many (11, 69%) emphasizing 'marked limitations'.

On longstay wards a majority of ward sisters (3, 75%) and staff nurses (4, 80%) acknowledged the requisite authority. Unit nurse managers concurred with this view. Many doctors (4, 67%) perceived limitations to nurses' authority. In contrast, all ward sisters (4, 100%) and staff nurses (5, 100%)

Table 6.3 Rating by nurses and other professionals of nurses' autonomy in district health authorities 1 and 2

Grade/profession	Acute medical (n=48)				Acute surgical (n=65)				Longstay (n=17)				
	Extremely free	Very free	Free	Not very free	Extremely free	Very free	Free	Not very free	Extremely free	Very free	Free	Not very free	n
Ward sister/charge nurse	2	2	2	–	1	5	5	–	–	1	1	2	21
Staff nurse	1	7	14	10	3	11	19	4	–	1	3	1	74
Unit nurse manager	1	1	–	–	1	1	–	–	–	2	–	–	6
Doctor	–	1	6	1	–	5	6	4	1	2	1	2	29
Total number of responses	4	11	22	11	5	22	30	8	1	6	5	5	130
Percentage of speciality responses	8	23	46	23	7	34	46	12	6	35	29	29	

perceived marked limitations to their freedom to act. Conversely, unit nurse managers perceived only 'some limitations', though 'no major constraints' on nurses' autonomy. Many doctors (4, 80%) perceived the autonomy of the ward sister and the staff nurse to be extremely limited in the execution of their job.

PERCEIVED IMPEDIMENTS

The main impediments or constraints perceived by ward sisters on the exercise of their authority and autonomy included the following. Doctors had prescriptive care, which prevented them using their expertise and discretion in the management of patient care. Nurse managers by their power and policies relating to resources and nursing practice sometimes substantially inhibited their freedom to make decisions, e.g. curtailing their ability to control and regulate the resourcing of their wards, particularly the number of staff and the direct effects of this on the care and wellbeing of the patients. They further limited their ability to regulate the workload and pressure on staff, for which they were accountable.

Staff nurses stated that impediments or constraints were similar to those identified by ward sisters, especially when they were in charge of the ward. In addition, little heed was paid to their views on patient care and ward management, innovation and change by some ward sisters, doctors and nurse managers. Innovative ideas were not encouraged or acted upon. They were obliged to work within narrow, ill-conceived guidelines on nursing practice put together by the Nursing Procedures Committee with no consultation at ward level. The constraints led to a lack of motivation and low morale, which affected their job satisfaction.

Unit and senior nurse managers perceived little, if any, constraints on nurses' authority and autonomy which would prevent them carrying out their prescribed responsibilities and duties, stating: 'Nurses are very free to manage their wards'. 'Staff think they are constrained tremendously; they use it as an excuse'.

In contrast to nurses' stated views on the extent of their authority, only a few (5%) regarded themselves as 'extremely free' to make decisions; the majority perceived their autonomy was severely constrained. There would appear to be contradictions built into the way nurses perceive their authority and autonomy. A comparison of Tables 6.1, 6.2 and Table 5.1, Chapter 5, reveal these contradictions.

OBJECTIVITY AND SUBJECTIVITY

The information provided by the study and especially identified in the foregoing tables suggests an objective and subjective dimension. The reality of nurses' objective, real authority and autonomy would appear to be based on the premise that these elements of the nurses' role are formally constructed, insofar as they are based on and influenced by the directives of management together with the associated rules and procedures, created and defined by management, over which many nurses have little or no control. These rules and procedures directly govern the job of the nurse and often may intentionally or unintentionally constrain them in doing their job as they would wish.

In practice, many nurses acknowledged little, if any, influence over nursing policy, resources and some nursing practices, which they said often were defined and regulated by a relatively unrepresentative, outmoded nursing procedures committee. They claimed there was little choice or flexibility in nursing practices, as policy was decided without any consultation with, or influence by, the ward team. They felt patronized when on rare occasions they were asked for their views by this committee, which they then ignored.

In contrast, nurses' subjective authority and autonomy appeared to be perceived by nurses as closely related to the ethic of their job, i.e. they were inherent in their emotional self, their sensitivity and intention to ensure that patients' needs were met, sometimes against heavy odds, over which from their responses they perceived themselves to have some influence; though the evidence of this study shows that they often failed in this endeavour.

The situation thus described poses many problems for nurses in the execution of their role; for nurse managers in the design, regulation and monitoring of nurses' work as encompassed in their job description; for nurse educators in the professional development of nurses in appropriate skills and knowledge, especially cognitive and effective skills, in order to improve nurses' confidence and assertiveness.

INTERRELATIONSHIP OF ROLE ELEMENTS

The elements of responsibility, authority, autonomy and accountability are much discussed (EEC, 1977, 1989; *Nurses, Midwives and Health Visitors Act 1979*; UKCC, 1986; RCN, 1988; UKCC, 1992a, 1992b) as prerequisites to enabling the effective performance of professional nurses in the management of patient care. The interrelationship of these elements and their relevance to the performance by nurses of their role is expressed by Batey and Lewis (1982) who perceived these elements as 'Inextricably related . . . Accountability is limited when nursing service can claim only authority of expert knowledge but not authority of position. Accountability is an exercise in futility and an experience in failure unless it is linked to nursing service's autonomy' (paras 6/7, p. 13). The schematic representation and interrelationship of these elements (Fig. 1) summarizes the links between the prescribed behaviours of nurses, the tasks which they perform, enabling or enacting their prescribed duties and responsibilities and the perceived subjectivity or objectivity of their authority and autonomy.

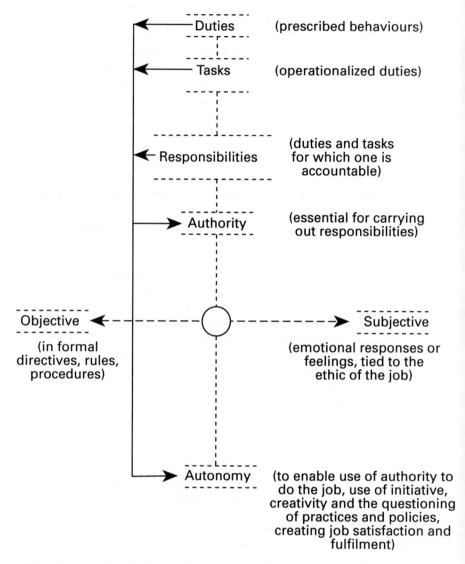

Fig. 1 Interrelationship between functions and elements of the nurses' role.

SUMMARY

There was little difference between individual nurses' perceptions and those of other professionals of nurses' lack of authority to manage their wards and care for their patients, i.e. to ensure its proper resourcing, plan workload, assess the workload, co-ordinate work, lead the ward team and ensure quality patient care. Most nurses in their responses perceived patient care as being 'the hands-on care of the patient' rather than viewing it in a broader perspective which embraced the total care of the patient, including ensuring their independence, comfort and general wellbeing. Professional nurses may be the victims of a system that tends to override and even annul their intellect and as a direct result causes them to behave sometimes in a passive non-assertive manner, thereby reducing their ability to make decisions in the performance of their role.

Some professionals are of the opinion that the authority and autonomy of newly registered nurses should be limited. However, is this realistic, given the situation described by many of these nurses? They claimed they were 'often thrown in at the deep end, without support, direction or counselling', when they were frequently anxious about the demands, responsibilities and organization of their new job. They were often 'left in charge' when they felt they had not been fully prepared for their role. This is further clarified in an RCN report (1988) which stated:

> Although changes in nurse education should mean that newly qualified nurses have learned how to practise professionally and be accountable, it is recognised that these nurses are still inexperienced and vulnerable. In their efforts to demonstrate capability and confidence as qualified nurses, they may be prone to make unwise judgments about the limits of their practice, particularly if left with insufficient support.
>
> *(Para. 3, p. 9)*

Even though this report was written five years ago and the educational initiatives of Project 2000 are *in situ*, on discussion with nurses and their managers, this traumatic situation was still found to exist. During the study, this situation frequently occurred. Newly qualified nurses had no preparation or induction for their new, demanding role as staff nurses.

Neither district health authority had a system of induction and support for newly appointed (first appointment) ward sisters, with some nurse managers accepting the situation as the norm, stating, 'You cannot teach ward management; the ward sister's job is best learned as you go along'. Irrespective of the merit of this statement, it was clear during discussions with the sisters that they felt it was necessary to have some induction and support. In the situation described, it is virtually asking the impossible of nurses to perform with confidence and assurance.

I would question the assertions of some officers of the nursing statutory and professional bodies, views shared to some extent by nurse managers, that the elements of role authority and autonomy are present but for reasons including 'traditional attitudes, compliance, submissiveness and lack of assertiveness' they lie dormant and in this way limit the impact of nurses on their role.

On discussion with nurses, some of whom had trained 10–20 years ago and many of whom had not undertaken further professional development, they often said the effects of what they referred to as traditional training, which encouraged respect for others, especially senior nurses and doctors, viewing other professionals as superior to themselves, reinforced by their perceived lack of training and professional status, paradoxically tarnished nurses' image and rendered them ineffective in the performance of their job.

In contrast, on observation, recently registered nurses (1–3 years), though admitting during interview problems that limited the effectiveness of their role, demonstrated less submissiveness and questioned practices even though they felt their opinions were not respected or heeded. On recent discussions with newly registered nurses, especially those undertaking training with Project 2000, they said their training encouraged them to be more assertive and questioning, but they felt fettered by the fact that 'we are afraid to rock the boat, or question too much; we would like to implement many of the new initiatives and practices learned during training but many of us only have fixed, short-term contracts which we hope to have renewed, so when our opinions are rejected, we tend to accept it. We have no alternative'.

Finally, the words of Rowbottom and Billis (1987) and Mayeroff (1971) echo some of these problems and set them in context. For example, Rowbottom and Billis get at the core of the problem of nurses' authority and autonomy when stating:

> A fundamental issue is the basic work level expected of any qualified nurse. Is the training which leads to statutory registration designed to produce fully-fledged professionals capable of making their own responses to complex situations? Or is it merely intended to produce a body of top-level technicians capable of carrying out a wide range of prescribed nursing procedures? . . . the position is greatly affected by whether the qualified nurse is seen by senior doctors as a subordinate technician or as a fellow professional.
>
> *(Paras 1/2, p. 114)*

Clearly, even though nurses' education until recent initiatives was not designed to produce 'fully-fledged professionals', nurses of necessity have had to be reactive and cope with the demands of complex situations in the performance of their role. The efficacy of these responses could be questioned in the absence of appropriate training and development. Developments under the aegis of Project 2000 will hopefully correct these anomalies and produce pro-active nurses, who are capable of effectively responding to complex situations with confidence and professionalism.

The concerns evidenced by nurses in the study regarding their subordination to other professionals will also be addressed, at least in theory, with current trends, i.e. equal named partners in the ward team, as long as other professionals are 'educated' about the new professional role of the nurse, and the nursing profession itself recognizes and understands the implications of this development and builds in its own support systems to enable this emancipation.

Much has been written over the past 25 years about nurses' authority and autonomy, often addressing the absence and/or limitations of these elements of role (Salmon, 1966; Hall, 1968; Engel, 1970; Mayeroff, 1971; Briggs, 1972; Merrison, 1979; RCN, 1982, 1988; Batey and Lewis, 1982; Rowbottom and Billis, 1987; DoH, Nursing Division, 1989; Audit Commission, 1991, 1992). The following chapter will discuss patients' needs, especially in light of the many acknowledged impediments to the nurses' role.

Patients: how well are their needs met?

BACKGROUND

As an introduction to the findings and to set them in context, the general statement by nurses and nurse managers is considered that, in addition to the sporadic use of different models of care, e.g. by Roper *et al.* (1985) and Orem (1985), the main framework or process used for meeting patients' needs was the 'nursing process' (the systematic, planned and evaluated care, which addresses patients' needs by use of an individual care plan). Nurses said that the nursing process was often difficult to sustain, due to inadequate staffing levels, which as a direct result prevented the lack of involvement of patients and their relatives in the care process.

This seems to be a defeatist attitude. The nursing process used as a positive step towards total patient care could have beneficial results, especially when there are staff shortages, e.g. involvement of the patient and relatives would decrease the mystique of some nursing practices, making the patient feel an important part of their own recovery, enabling a measure of independence, reducing the time patients have to ask repeated questions because no one tells them what is happening and furthering a better nurse/patient/relative relationship.

DEFINITION OF TERMS

The following definitions are used in the discussion of patients' needs.

Patients' needs
'Requirements for the maintenance of patients' wellbeing' (Kraegel *et al.*, 1972).

Caring
In essence, meeting patients' needs. In the context of needs Mayeroff (1971) states 'To care for someone I must know what his needs are' (para. 1, p. 9).
Evaluation of care
Comprises a sequence of logical steps which includes selecting and specifying standards; developing the means by which the specified standards may be judged to have been achieved; the collection and analysis of such judgments, and the reporting and feedback of results' (RCN, 1980, para. 42, pp. 10/11).
Standard of care
The desired and achievable level of performance corresponding with a criterion against which actual performance is compared (Block, 1977).
A criterion
The value-free name of a variable believed or known to be a relevant indicator of the quality of patient care (Block, 1977).
Quality of care
The degree of excellence of the care provided including the integrity, sensitivity and humanity of nursing activities and interventions which are done with interest, enthusiasm, enlightenment and interaction with patients which must include patient participation and consultation (Bowman, 1986).
Nursing standards
How well an individual nurse meets an individual patient's needs (RCN, 1981, para. 3, p. 2).

The system used to organize the daily care of patients on most wards included the use of two models of care. The Roper model includes 12 activities of daily living and was found by nurses who used it to adapt readily to meeting the needs of most patients, especially stroke patients. Orem's model emphasizes patient involvement in care and rehabilitation and was found to be particularly useful by the nurses, as a framework to care for patients who required special training with, for example, incontinence and colostomy/ileostomy.

The team approach to the care of patients was favoured by three ward sisters; two or three nurses were used in the team, depending on staffing levels. Each team had a mix of grades, e.g. staff nurse, enrolled nurse, nursing student and care assistant (nursing auxiliary). This system was found to be especially useful in enabling the continuity of care for patients as well as enhancing and improving nurses' information on patients' problems and enabling the leadership and improved learning by nurses. Despite the identification of these models and their stated advantages, a number of ward sisters (43%) and staff nurses (54%) said that because of various impediments, notably staff shortages, a task-related approach to care was used.

Some ward sisters (14%) and staff nurses (28%) said that the system approach to the care of the patient varied considerably. In this respect, the influences underlined by them which prevented the regular use of a systematic approach to care and, as a direct result, the adoption of a task-related approach included inadequate staffing levels coupled with a heavy workload, clinically and administratively. Many professional nurses, ward sisters (68%) and staff nurses (75%) agreed that the task-related work could be done quicker as it did not involve the patient.

'The nursing process' was frequently alluded to, though virtually wholly in the context of its added burden of administration, e.g. notation of patients' history, care plan formulation and record keeping. Only two (10%) ward sisters and five (7%) staff nurses said they used the nursing process fully and often, to care for their patients.

On observation there appeared to be no one system used but a mixture of different systems and approaches, none of which could be identified in its entirety. There was a combination of individual and team approach systems of care. These often 'broke down' due to the oft repeated 'lack of time; staff shortages'. Attempts by ward sisters and staff nurses were impeded by the movement of staff to supply for shortages on other wards. They were concerned about their inability to control resources, especially the use of temporary staff, as this reduced stability insofar as advanced planning was concerned. This is echoed in a recent report (Seccombe and Ball, 1992), which states: 'twelve percent of hospital nurses were unable to classify the mode of care delivery they currently worked with' (para. 6.1, p. 64). Virtually all nurses agreed it was impossible, because of many impediments, to care for their patients as people with individual needs, in a professional manner.

The care of patients on observation and based on responses of many nurses tended to be very mechanized, i.e. ritualized through the performance of tasks and procedures, with little patient involvement. The reasons frequently given for this ritualized, mechanized care included an inordinate nursing and administrative workload; rapid turnover of patients; frequent transfer of patients between wards, due to shortage of beds; and the regular practice of employing agency nurses, some of whom were said to be unskilled in the clinical needs of patients.

The involvement of the patients in their care, together with their relatives, where practicable, is deemed to be central to the 'nursing process'. Yet in reality the responses of ward sisters, staff nurses, doctors and some nurse managers indicated little, if any, patient-relative involvement in patients' care. Many (65%) nurses, especially staff nurses, stated that because time was at a premium, and nurses were few, the inclusion of patients and their relatives in the care programme proved an inhibitor to their work.

Some (33%) nurse managers perceived the role of the patient as passive, being informed of their care, but doubted if they should be involved. They said that many nurses saw the role of the patient as a passive one; nurses tended to undermine the independence of the patient. However, most (66%) nurse managers agreed that patients should be involved in their care programme.

The responses of most nurses (85%), confirmed by the observation of nurses' behaviours, indicated that little real discussion and negotiation took place during doctors' ward rounds, other than nurses informing doctors of patients' progress and special occurrences relating to the condition of the patients, and doctors requesting information about the patients or giving instructions to nurses about patients' future treatment. The information provided by nurses to doctors during formal and/or informal ward rounds included patients' medication, mobility, diet, sleep patterns, change of treatment and discharge. Many (55%) staff nurses and some (10%) ward sisters said 'some doctors, especially consultants, prescribed patients' care'. Many doctors (30%) said 'nurses are unable to make decisions about basic clinical practices which require little skill, e.g. the removal of a nasogastric tube when no further aspirate was being produced, and wound care, and often to their annoyance referred these situations to them for a decision'.

During observation there was little evidence of negotiation on patients' care. Doctors' instructions to nurses were evident. There appeared to be a fine line between treatment and care. Normally one would expect an agreed/negotiated policy on the role of the professional nurse and the role of the doctor within the ward. However, from observation and nurses' comments it was evident that the doctors' role, especially for registrars and house officers, encroached upon the role of the nurse. This became a problem area between nursing and medical staff, with ward sisters (38%) stating 'Doctors interfered with and sometimes influenced established care regimes and would not accept our views and advice on patient care'. Staff nurses (51%) said that the approach to patient care by some doctors, including consultants, was old-fashioned and prescriptive insofar as it did not relate to current and informed nursing practice, e.g. the use of dressings as opposed to plastic sealant. When questioned about these differing views on patient care, especially where the medical view prevailed, the nurses' responses appeared to be defeatist, with the claim: 'We have no redress; we lack the authority to do anything about it'.

DIRECT 'HANDS-ON' PATIENT CARE

In the main, based on the responses of nurses, even though they wanted to be involved directly with the care of their patients, most care was given by enrolled nurses, nursing students and care assistants. This point is made in a recent report by the Audit Commission (1992) which describes 'The ward sister as clinical nurse, struggling to retain a foothold in patient care, at odds at what she feels to be the illegitimate calls on her time that take her away from patients and students' (para. 69, p. 31).

The majority of nurses (ward sisters 95%, staff nurses 98%) said that their principal desire was to be close to their patients but regrettably, often they were prevented from doing so by other duties and tasks, central to which was the much repeated vast amount of 'paperwork' embodied in ward administra-

Table 7.1 Rating by nurses and other professionals of the extent to which nurses could ensure the wellbeing of patients, in district health authorities 1 and 2, for all clinical specialities

Grade/profession	Completely	To a reasonable extent	On the whole, Yes	Not usually	Impossible	n
Ward sister/charge nurse	33	38	29	0	0	21
Staff nurse	41	47	12	0	0	74
Unit nurse manager	50	0	50	0	0	6
Senior nurse managers	50	0	50	0	0	2
Doctors	14	38	41	0	7	29
Officer of statutory body	0	0	50	50	0	2
Officer of professional body	0	0	0	100	0	1

tion, including that associated with the nursing process, which was seen by many professionals, including doctors, as being a ritual in procedure and administration.

How did the various groups within the sample respond to questions relating to the safety and wellbeing of patients, ensuring safe standards of practice through supervision of staff, setting nursing standards and evaluating nursing care and generally ensuring for patients a consistently high, professional standard of care? Tables 7.1, 7.2 and 7.3 summarize the responses of nurses and other professionals to these questions. They key to the rating of responses is as follows:

Completely:	Always
To a reasonable extent:	Most times
On the whole, Yes:	It depends, sometimes
Not usually:	Seldom, if at all
Impossible:	Never

HOW DID PATIENTS PERCEIVE THEIR NEEDS WERE MET?

Patients were selected for interview following initial discussion with the nurse in charge of the ward as to their medical status, i.e. patients too ill to participate were excluded. Every fourth patient (approximately 20%) on each ward where nurses were observed was invited to answer questions relating to their stay on the ward, particularly on how they perceived their care. A total of 81 patients from medical (32), surgical (42) and longstay (7) wards were

Table 7.2 Rating by nurses and other professionals of the extent to which nurses could ensure safe standards of practice, in district health authorities 1 and 2, for all clinical specialities

Grade/profession	Completely	To a reasonable extent	On the whole, Yes	Not usually	Impossible	n
Ward sister/charge nurse	48	29	18	0	5	21
Staff nurse	49	41	10	0	0	74
Nurse manager	0	67	33	0	0	6
Senior nurse manager	0	50	50	0	0	2
Doctor	7	28	48	10	7	29
Officer of statutory body	0	0	50	50	0	2
Officer of professional body	0	100	0	0	0	1

Table 7.3 Rating by nurses and other professionals of the extent to which nurses could ensure the adequate resourcing of their wards, in district health authorities 1 and 2, for all clinical specialities

Grade/profession	Completely	To a reasonable extent	On the whole, Yes	Not usually	Impossible	n
Ward sister/charge nurse	0	19	38	33	10	21
Staff nurse	7	24	45	15	9	74
Unit nurse manager	9	33	0	67	0	6
Senior nurse manager	0	0	50	50	0	2
Doctor	3	0	17	17	63	29
Officer of statutory body	0	0	50	50	0	2
Officer of professional body	0	0	0	0	100	1

interviewed. One patient refused to participate, preferring not to discuss her care. There were 41 and 40 patients respectively from District Health Authority 1 and 2.

Patients' needs were identified essentially during the pre-pilot and pilot study, the patients identifying what they perceived as important. The interview schedule was evaluated in terms of its appropriateness. An interview manual was kept so that any rephrasing or rewording of questions was consistently maintained. The total time taken for all interviews was approximately 17 hours; each patient interview was approximately 13 minutes.

Patient dependency levels on wards where interviews were conducted fell into two categories, high and intermediate, for both districts (Table 7.4). A

Table 7.4 Observed patient dependency levels for 81 patients in three types of ward

Dependency	Male	Female	Total
Acute medical			
High	5	8	13
Intermediate	9	10	19
Acute surgical			
High	6	7	13
Intermediate	13	16	29
Longstay			
High	3	4	7

five-point scale was used to determine to what extent patients perceived their needs were met (Table 7.5). The key to the rating of responses is as follows:

Great extent:	Regularly, daily
Fair extent:	Often, but not regularly
Some extent:	Occasionally, inadequately
Inadequately:	Seldom, if at all
Not applicable:	Sometimes, for medical reasons

COMMENT

From the responses of nurses and patients it is evident that nurses were unable to ensure the complete wellbeing of the patient and were not always able to provide the standard and quality of care at a professional level which patients rightfully expect, in their endeavour to meet the needs of their patients. Patients' perceptions identified many shortcomings. In fact, out of a total of 135 respondents to the question of whether patients' needs were met, only a fraction of the entire sample of nurses, nurse managers, doctors and officers of the statutory and professional bodies responded in the affirmative.

Given this result, how did patients respond to their care and the meeting of their needs? The number of patients ($n = 81$) who were satisfied with their care was 57 (70%); the number dissatisfied with their care was 24 (30%). However,

Table 7.5 Rating by 81 patients of the extent to which they perceived their needs were met

	Great extent	Fair extent	Some extent	Inad- equately	Not applicable
Physical needs					
1. Comfort (general)	82.72	9.88	3.70	3.70	–
2. Elimination (bladder and bowels)	86.42	1.23	–	12.35	–
3. Food	80.25	11.11	1.23	7.41	–
4. Pain relief	75.31	1.23	1.23	2.47	19.75
5. Personal hygiene	92.59	–	–	1.23	6.17
6. Rest	44.44	12.35	16.05	27.16	–
7. Safety	96.30	1.23	1.23	1.23	–
8. Sleep	37.04	13.58	17.28	32.10	–
Emotional needs					
1. Reduction of apprehension	40.74	24.69	14.81	18.52	1.23
2. Reduction of anxiety	39.51	23.46	14.81	20.99	1.23
3. Advice (health education)	40.74	11.11	14.81	29.63	3.70
4. Explanation (about treatments)	33.33	13.58	17.28	34.57	1.23
5. Fear reduction	38.75	21.25	13.75	22.50	3.75
6. Information (care, progress, ward procedure)	33.33	9.88	19.75	37.04	–
7. Security	92.59	6.17	–	1.23	–
8. Sympathy	87.65	7.41	2.47	2.47	–
9. Kindness (by ward staff)	95.06	4.94	–	–	–
10. Informal talking by staff to patient	40.74	12.35	24.69	22.22	–
Social needs					
1. Confidentiality (condition)	86.42	3.70	1.23	7.41	1.24
2. Dignity (self-respect)	64.20	19.75	9.88	6.17	–
3. Friendliness (ward staff)	95.06	3.70	1.23	–	–
4. Identity (individual)	77.78	13.58	6.17	2.47	–
5. Independence (exercise of reasonable freedom)	83.95	12.35	1.23	1.23	1.23
6. Likes and dislikes	56.25	30.0	7.50	3.75	2.5
7. Privacy	23.75	35.0	23.75	17.5	–
Spiritual needs					
1. Hospital chaplain	29.63	4.94	4.94	41.98	18.52
2. Religious service	6.25	1.25	2.5	5.0	85.0

even though a high percentage of patients indicated satisfaction with their overall care, many of these patients rated some of their needs inadequately met (Table 7.6).

The main elements of satisfaction deemed essential during their stay in hospital were perceived by patients to include being well cared for; kindness of staff; being given information about their progress and ward routine, i.e. what

Table 7.6 Patients' perceptions ($n = 31$, 38%) of how their needs were met

Need	Great extent	Fair extent	Some extent	Inadequately	n
Health education	0	0	12	24	36
Visit by chaplain	0	0	4	33	37
Explanation (care and treatment)	0	0	15	28	43
Fear reduction	0	0	9	25	34
Information (ward procedure/ progress)	0	0	16	29	45
Privacy	0	0	19	13	32
Rest	0	0	12	21	33
Sleep	0	0	13	25	38
Talking informally	0	0	20	17	37

to do and what not to do; receiving prompt attention; relief of pain; comfort; being talked to informally when doctors and nurses were near them or treating them; being helped to understand their predicament; being treated as a human being; privacy; being able to talk to nurses and doctors without fear of being overheard by other patients. The last was frequently not met.

The main elements of patients' dissatisfaction during their stay in hospital was perceived by them to include lack of privacy, especially when they were distressed or undergoing toileting and intimate procedures; lack of rest and sleep, sometimes being awakened at 6.30 AM, being given a cup of tea and asked to go back to sleep; lack of dignity, e.g. some patients complained they were asked about 'waterworks, everybody heard the answer'; lack of confidentiality: 'screens inadequate . . . could hear information about other patients, if you wanted to . . . everyone seems to know what's wrong with you'; not being able to get attention, e.g. being admitted at 2.30 PM and not being seen by anybody before 7.45 PM; lack of ward cleanliness; small dayroom, intended for visitors only, not patients; loss of independence: 'they sometimes do too much for you' (probably because of task-related approach); and not enough visits or no visit by the hospital chaplain. One ward sister said she had reported this matter to nursing management but with little effect.

Even though the above reasons were given as direct causes of patients' dissatisfaction, many patients additionally said there was a lack of information and explanation about their condition, which aggravated their fears and worries, particularly heightening their dissatisfaction. In the main, younger patients (20–40-year age group) commented more openly and vigorously than the middle-aged or elderly group on the inadequacies of their care.

In this context, this was exemplified in a recent research study (Breemhaar, Visser and Kleijnen, 1990), where it was stated that 'Elderly patients were more satisfied than younger patients with the more measured aspects of treatment, care and support during their hospital stay' (para. 1, p. 1381).

PERCEIVED IMPEDIMENTS
IN THE DELIVERY OF PATIENT CARE

Nurses acknowledged many impediments which they said prevented them from caring for their patients as they would wish. Many of these impediments have already been acknowledged in the text and can be summarized as manpower related, workload related, time related (Table 7.7).

These stated impediments were evident during periods of observed nurses' behaviour but need to be questioned as to their validity, for example, the way the workload was organized on the basis of expediency with more regard given to the needs of nurses than to needs of patients and without proper utilization of nursing skills, e.g. staff nurses doing tea rounds while auxiliaries did blood pressures. Sisters and staff nurses were doing clerical work while the ward clerks seemed to be duplicating this effort. There appeared to be very little organization and informed delegation.

This situation is acknowledged in general terms by the Audit Commission (1992) which states: 'what distinguishes the wards that are succeeding in achieving greater continuity and more patient-centred care from others, is that they manage to use all their resources, including clerical to release nursing time for patients' (para. 22, p. 15).

Patient dependency produced a workload that was often difficult to address, because of the inadequate nature (the mix) and number of staff. Many nurses and doctors highlighted as major impediments to the proper care of patients the administrative workload, which often kept nurses office-bound and limited their ability to supervise subordinate nurses and untrained staff. It was stated that this situation was often compounded by the regular use of agency nurses, trained and untrained, who were frequently perceived to lack the necessary skills and knowledge of the different clinical specialities to which they were allocated. This was compounded by the fact that ward sisters had no choice or control over their allocation to their ward and it only served to increase the workload, as time was spent informing and inducting the nurse on ward practices and procedures. They further complained that after induction and time spent, there was no firm attachment to a ward as 'agency staff seem to be randomly allocated'.

One district health authority reduced the possibility of this mismatch by employing all newly registered nurses, who otherwise were unable to secure employment, as their own bank nurses. This solution, according to the nurse manager, 'obviated the problems encouraged and encountered by the random employment of agency nurses'. Initially this seemed to be a reasonable idea, but on reflection and examination it only served as an expedient, as these

Table 7.7 Impediments perceived by nurses and other professionals to the meeting of patients' needs, in district health authorities 1 and 2, for all clinical specialities

Need	Perceived impediments
Belonging	Rapid patient turnover; lack of time; size of ward
Comfort	Condition of patient; unsuitable/unsatisfactory or lack of hospital beds, mattresses or chairs
Confidentiality	Inadequate curtains; no facilities to discuss in private, doctors tend to discuss patients, and talk to them from the foot of the bed; extended family; too many people have access to patients' information
Dignity (self respect)	Lack of facilities, e.g. bed curtains, and inadequate toilet facilities
Emotional needs (reassurance, reduction of fear and anxiety)	Workload; no time; inadequate staffing levels
Friendliness	No impediments were identified
Identity (recognition as a person, individual)	In the main met satisfactorily. However, impediments identified included many admissions; rapid turnover of patients; labelling of patients, e.g. 'that operation', 'number X', 'bed X'
Information (care, progress, ward procedure)	No time to discuss matters with patients; sometimes only little information known about patient's condition
Independence	Quicker to do things oneself; hospital tradition
Likes and dislikes (within reason)	In the main accommodated quite satisfactorily
Pain relief	This was mostly met satisfactorily. However, the difficulty of assessing pain level was identified, due largely to lack of training of nurses in pain assessment and pain relief
Personal hygiene	Shortage of staff; lack of time
Physical (food, drink, bodily protection)	Food and drink were met well; reasons given for the inadequacy of bodily protection were as for safety
Privacy	Thin curtains; no real facilities; Nightingale-type wards
Rest	Ward practices and procedures, e.g. awakened at 6.30 AM; noisy patients; ward rounds; admission of patients at night; vicinity of ward to noise, e.g. accident and emergency unit
Safety	Inadequate supervision of staff; difficulty in supervision of patients all the time; staffing levels; much work done by untrained, inexperienced and unqualified staff
Sleep	Similar reasons were given to those for rest
Religious practice (ensuring a visit by the hospital chaplain; attending religious services)	Some patients indicated the non-applicability of religious service. No reason was given for infrequency of visits. However, on talking to patients, many indicated a desire to see the chaplain. One patient was disturbed because the chaplain visited the patient in the next bed, but did not speak to her. One ward sister reported non-visits by the chaplain to nursing management
Talking to patient informally	Workload; staffing levels

nurses were still used to fill gaps when there were staff shortages, and received no further staff development in special skills to meet the requirements of the wards to which they were allocated, or to enable them to further their professional career.

The shortage of material resources was especially emphasized by many (85%) staff nurses and some (40%) ward sisters to operate against sound clinical practice, and they cited the unavailability of syringes (had to be borrowed from other wards), sphygmomanometers (frequently broken) and the lack of hoists and monitoring equipment. The situation was further compounded by difficulty experienced, especially by staff nurses when in charge, in getting the services of social workers, occupational therapists and physiotherapists when required to assist their patients. This situation was particularly underlined by staff working on longstay wards and some surgical wards, one nurse stating that some doctors said the provision of these services served little purpose.

It is clear that these findings are due to many causes, which are highlighted in a DHSS report (Wright-Warren, 1986), which stated:

> The proportion of qualified staff varied considerably between the specialities. It was higher in the high dependency and lower in the longstay areas; lowest of all in wards for people with mental handicap. And, there was considerable variation in staffing levels between and within all specialities. Variations in cost tended to follow variations in staffing levels; skill mix had less effect, mainly because of narrow pay differentials and the way in which nursing staff costs were calculated. Small wards and units tended to be more costly in terms of staffing. In the longstay areas this was partly because they often had the most dependent or disturbed patients.
>
> *(Paras 5/6, p. vi)*

Many of the findings, e.g. blurred lines of communication, early awakening of patients and nurses' time on clerical duties, were amplified in a recent Audit Commission report (1991) which states:

> Nursing care needs to become more tailored to the needs of individual patients. Patients often do not know which nurse or group of nurses is looking after them, or who is able to give them information about their treatment. A majority of patients would prefer not to be woken so early (5 and 6 AM), and yet it is common practice on many wards. Many nurses spend over a quarter of their time on clerical and housekeeping tasks.
>
> *(Paras 1/4/42, pp. 1/2/8)*

Even though some needs were not met to the satisfaction of patients, most patients (70%) on interview said they were 'satisfied generally with their care', which they associated with 'sympathetic and caring staff, and getting well'. When patients were asked what caused their stress or disquiet during their stay in hospital, the majority (80%) included in their responses: lack of information; ward practices including being awakened early in the morning, which they acknowledged had little to do with their wellbeing; strange environment; missing home and family; loneliness, often with no one to talk to; not knowing what was going to happen, 'you get embarrassed, having to always ask for information such as the results of tests or examinations; even though the nurses must know you are anxious, they don't give results very quickly'; fear of operation and anaesthetic, and not knowing whether they would ever return home. From this information it is clear that the problems that confront patients during their stay in hospital are often many and great, and require sensitivity and action by nurses, doctors and other professionals.

Many ward sisters (75%) and staff nurses (65%) said they could not satisfactorily meet patients' needs, including those of belonging (making them feel 'at home'), dignity, information, independence, privacy, rest and sleep, talking informally to patients and treating patients as individuals. Some ward sisters (20%) and staff nurses (10%) said they had difficulty sometimes in ensuring the personal hygiene of patients. 'There are not enough handbasins, bathrooms, hoists, etc., and sometimes you need two or more nurses to deal with certain patients, and the staff are not available'.

In contrast, unit nurse managers (83%) stated that most of the needs identified were met completely, and to their satisfaction. However, senior nurse managers said 'Many nurses in our view are unable to meet adequately the needs of rest, sleep and communication with patients, because of ward practices, including frequent interruptions by many doctors, e.g. during the night, mealtimes, etc.'. On questioning and observation of doctors about this, the situation thus described was rationalized: 'Because of time and inordinate workload, it is unavoidable'.

Doctors, in the main, perceived that most patients' needs were inadequately met, especially emphasizing those of individuality, emotional reassurance, information, pain relief, independence, privacy, rest, sleep and safety.

Officers of the statutory and professional bodies perceived that patients' needs, which were probably inadequately met, included those of confidentiality, independence, rest and sleep, safety and privacy.

Many of the views expressed underline the nurses' difficulty, for different reasons, in being able to meet patients' needs fully.

The new initiatives, *The Patients' Charter* (DoH, 1991) and the *NHS and Community Care Act 1990*, will require nurses to change their attitude and realize that the service is now patient-led, and not the dictatorial service it has been in the past. Patients have a right to have their needs met and nurses must ensure that this obligation on their part is satisfied. *The Patients' Charter* states that 'Charter rights are guaranteed' (para. 1, p. 19). Recently, health authorities have been preparing strategy programmes for contracts and have realized that they have never met the needs, even to a reasonable extent, of patients with a sensory handicap. Of hospital attenders, 17% are people with a sensory handicap, yet they are not included in *A Strategy for Nursing* (DoH Nursing Division, 1989). It is not enough to talk about the delivery of quality services to all patients, as embodied in *The Patients' Charter* (para. 1, p. 13) and simultaneously neglect to confront the issues relating to the care of patients with a sensory handicap.

There is a failure of society in general, and health service personnel in particular, to recognize that people with a disability and/or handicap are not a homogeneous group, and that everyone has the potentiality to become a person with a disability. The key areas that give rise to concern are lack of disability awareness training of all staff and lack of access, not only into a building, but also to information in formats that can be accessed, e.g. Braille, large print, audio cassettes, British sign language and appropriate telephone systems. Proposals and steps to remedy the situation of addressing patients' needs will be discussed in Chapter 9. *The Patients' Charter* makes it clear that a number of the findings in the research relating to meeting patients' needs would most certainly be a breach of the guarantee of charter rights.

Much has been published relating to patients' needs, underlining the inadequacy and problems in their being met and the obligations that nurses have in meeting needs (Powell, 1966; WHO, 1966; Briggs, 1972; Merrison, 1979; Orem, 1985; Roper *et al.*, 1985; Wright-Warren, 1986; Moores and Thompson, 1986; DoH Nursing Division, 1989; Kitson, 1990; DoH, 1991; Audit Commission, 1991, 1992; UKCC, 1992a, 1992b; NHS Management Executive, 1992).

The function of nursing management is to match necessary and available resources to patient needs, needs which are never static but vary according to individual patients. The provision of nursing services and nursing care must always be directly related to meeting those needs so that nursing becomes patient-centred.

The following chapter discusses how nurses perceive that the many inadequacies and shortcomings identified contribute to their stress.

8	# Nurses' stress: parallels with other professionals

BACKGROUND

This chapter discusses nurses' stress as unfolded by them and often commented on by other professionals during many interviews and periods of observed behaviour, and its parallels with other professionals. Nurses' stress, its nature and causes, has been much discussed over the last two centuries. One hundred and fifty years ago, a national newspaper made the following statement:

> Hospital nurses have for the last year or two, been the victims of much unmerited abuse – they have their faults, but most of these may be laid to the want of proper treatment. Lectured by committees, preached at by chaplains, scowled on by treasurers and stewards, scolded by matrons, sworn at by surgeons, bullied by dressers; grumbled at and abused by patients; insulted if old and ill-favoured; talked flippantly to if middle-aged and good humoured; tempted and seduced if young and well-looking; they are what any woman might be exposed to the same influences, – meek, pious, saucy, careless, drunken, according to the circumstances and temperament; but mostly attentive and rarely unkind.
>
> *(The Times, 1857)*

Throughout this century a steady though ever increasing commentary emphasizing the disabling effects has centred on the incidence, causes, problems and preventive factors of nurses' stress, including that by Marshall (1980) who states that the 'Nurse's role implicitly is chiefly one of handling stress. She is a focus for the stress of the patient, relatives and doctor, as well as her own' (para. 3, p. 21). However, there are many permutations of this opinion which could be debated, e.g. a nurse not doing her job well or sensitively could put further stress on the patient or indeed the doctor.

The effects of stress on the person and the organization are many and well catalogued. They include those of fatigue, helplessness, lack of concentration, absenteeism, and physical, emotional and mental debility leading to the phenomenon of burnout, where the nurse is drained of all energy and which constitutes a serious state of health. In addition, the organization in which the nurse works may be affected by attrition rates and absenteeism. The compound effect of these can produce a potential source of harm for the individual who is stressed, patients and colleagues. The effect of unrecognized and/or untreated stress on the nurse can lead to accidents to him/herself and/or others, including patients, due to lack of concentration, lack of judgement and lack of self esteem; for example, errors may occur in the checking and administration of drugs.

A worrying consequence of untreated nurses' stress is the potential last resort of a dependence on alcohol and drugs and sometimes, in extreme cases, suicide. Even though there is no tangible evidence or numbers available to link drug and alcohol abuse to nurses' stress, it is understood from discussions with nurses' welfare services that a number of cases summoned to appear before the UKCC Disciplinary Committee are drug or alcohol related.

During the study, when nurses were asked how they dealt with their stress, they replied: 'Have a drink'; 'Have a good cry'; 'Talk to friends' and/or 'Discuss with family'; 'Have splitting headaches, so have to take analgesics'. During discussion, many nurses said 'Living alone in flats doesn't help; you have no one to discuss things with' and 'there is no named person in the hospital that can help; we have an occupational health service but it's mainly for physical problems'.

Following the disclosure by many nurses (ward sisters 71%, $n = 15$ and staff nurses 91%, $n = 67$) of their stress, often perceived by them to be in excess of what they regarded to be tolerable, it was decided to further investigate the existence/extent of nurses' stress, together with the provision of support facilities at hospital/district/national level.

The extent of the problem of stress in general is discussed in a recent report, which states: 'Stress costs the country £7 billion every year. Stress accounts for 80 million lost working days every year. Yet, only 12% of companies have a mental health policy' (MIND, 1992).

The activities especially perceived by nurses as stress-provoking included workload, staffing levels, attempting to ensure standards of care, demanding responsibilities, lack of autonomy and in particular their lack of freedom to make decisions about the resourcing of their wards and the care of their patients, lack of career prospects and lack of job security. (For details of source, frequency and intensity of nurses' stress see Table 8.1.)

Many ward sisters and staff nurses, on interview, described a stressful role, graphically describing the undermining, disabling and generally disruptive effects of stress on themselves insofar as they were often tired, worn-out and unable to have a proper social life. Also, many nurses said that as a result of

Table 8.1 Source, frequency and intensity of nurses' stress

Source	Frequency	Intensity
Ward sister/charge nurse		
Role/job related		
1. Constant interruptions, e.g. doctors, relatives, telephone	Regular	Very stressful
2. Lack of professional status	Regular	Stressful
3. Workload (inordinate, various brief and fragmented)	Regular	Very stressful
4. Administration, paperwork	Regular	Stressful
5. Conflicting demands	Regular	Stressful
6. Multiple responsibilities	Regular	Very stressful
7. Inability to meet some responsibilities, e.g. safety of patient	Regular	Greatly stressful
8. Poor working conditions	Often	Stressful
9. Inadequate information	Often	Stressful
10. Being kept informed by management of new events and change	Often	Stressful
11. Frequent change, no time to adjust	Often	Stressful
12. Lack of feedback on performance	Regular	Stressful
13. Interference by nurse manager	Sometimes	Very stressful
14. Lack of real authority	Constant	Stressful
15. Lack of autonomy	Constant	Stressful
16. Little job satisfaction	Constant	Stressful
17. Lack of educational up-dating	Constant	Stressful
18. Low morale	Constant	Stressful
19. Lack of counselling and support	Constant	Stressful
Patient-related		
1. Transfer of patients to and from other wards	Regular	Stressful
2. High dependency – very ill patients	Regular	Very stressful
3. Emergencies	Regular	Stressful
4. Not enouth time to talk to patients	Regular	Stressful
5. Need to maintain standards and quality of care that are professionally accepted	Regular	Extremely stressful
6. Inability to care for patients professionally	Regular	Very stressful
Resource-related		
1. Lack of resources	Regular	Very stressful
2. Lack of facilities (toilets, hoists)	Regular	Very stressful
3. Lack of trained/experienced staff	Regular	Very stressful
4. Use of unqualified/inexperienced staff	Regular	Very stressful
5. Use of agency nurses	Regular	Very stressful
6. No control over resources	Regular	Stressful
7. Undue reliance on nursing students and nursing auxiliaries for patient care	Regular	Stressful
Doctor–related		
1. Many 'mini' rounds	Regular	Stressful
2. Many consultants and registrars servicing the ward	Regular	Stressful

Table 8.1—*continued*

Source	Frequency	Intensity
3. 'Monitoring' junior doctors' work (often requested by consultant)	Regular	Stressful
4. Conflict in approach to patient care	Sometimes	Very stressful
Task-related		
1. Coping with patients' relatives	Regular	Very stressful
2. Ensuring work gets done	Regular	Very stressful
3. Inability to nurse patients, because of administrative duties	Regular	Very stressful
4. Not always able to do things properly	Regular	Very stressful
5. Constant interruptions, e.g. telephone ringing	Regular	Very stressful
6. Lack of opportunity to give individualized care	Regular	Very stressful
7. Variety, brevity and fragmentation	Regular	Very stressful
Educational/vocational-related		
Difference between educational preparation, personal aspirations and the reality of the job, i.e. patient-oriented; job is essentially managerial/administratively oriented	Regular	Stressful
Staff nurse		
Role/job-related		
1. Lack of preparation for job, inadequacy of educational development	Regular	Extremely stressful
2. Constant interruptions, e.g. doctors, telephone, patients, other nurses	Regular	Extremely stressful
3. Workload	Regular	Stressful
4. Lack of status	Regular	Very stressful
5. Lack of professional acknowledgement	Regular	Stressful
6. Managerial and administrative duties (not being prepared)	Regular	Very stressful
7. Teaching of nurses	Regular	Stressful
8. Too many duties (overload)	Regular	Very stressful
9. Excessive responsibility	Regular	Very stressful
10. Lack of feedback on performance (given only on complaints)	Regular	Stressful
11. Deputizing for sister	Regular	Stressful
12. Lack of 'real' authority	Regular	Stressful
13. Lack of freedom to introduce new ideas (creativity stunted/ignored)	Often	Stressful
14. Conflicting demands of role	Often	Stressful
15. Worrying ('Have things been done properly?')	Regular	Very stressful
16. Being 'thrown in at the deep end' (newly qualified nurses)	Regular	Very stressful
17. Lack of recognition of work done (never praised)	Regular	Stressful
18. Lack of support and understanding of job	Regular	Stressful
19. Low morale	Regular	Stressful

Table 8.1—*continued*

Source	Frequency	Intensity
20. Lack of counselling/support	Regular	Stressful
21. Frequent change, with little preparation	Regular	Stressful
Patient-related		
1. Dealing with emergency admissions	Regular	Stressful
2. Not enough time to talk to patients, to reassure them	Regular	Stressful
3. Trying to maintain standards of care	Regular	Very stressful
4. Unable to care for patients professionally (as one would wish)	Regular	Very stressful
5. Being unable to ensure safety of patient	Regular	Very stressful
Resource-related		
1. Lack of resources	Regular	Very stressful
2. Lack of trained, experienced staff	Regular	Stressful
3. Undue reliance on nursing students/nursing auxiliaries for patient care	Regular	Stressful
4. Use of agency nurses	Regular	Stressful
5. No control over resources	Regular	Stressful
6. Constant borrowing of equipment	Regular	Stressful
Doctor-related		
1. Many 'mini' ward rounds	Regular	Stressful
2. Dealing with doctors' ward rounds (emphasized by newly registered nurses)	Regular	Stressful
3. Conflict in approach to patient care	Sometimes	Stressful
4. Outmoded ideas on patient care and treatment (nursing)	Sometimes	Stressful
Task-related		
1. Coping with patients' relatives	Sometimes	Stressful
2. Coping with bereavement (little training/counselling given)	Sometimes	Stressful
3. Coping with terminally ill patients	Often	Stressful
4. Trying to get the work done	Regular	Very stressful
5. Caring for patients prior to abortion	Regular	Very stressful
6. Unable to nurse patients because of too much managerial/administrative work	Regular	Stressful
7. Not always able to do things properly	Regular	Stressful
8. Liaising with many people	Regular	Stressful
9. Ritualized impersonal care	Regular	Stressful
10. No time to think or work things out properly	Regular	Stressful
11. Many interruptions (doctors' visits)	Regular	Stressful
Educational/vocational-related		
Difference between educational preparation, personal aspirations and the reality of the job, i.e. patient-oriented; job is essentially managerial/administratively oriented	Regular	Stressful

stress, they felt their job suffered. This is evidenced by Gray-Toft and Anderson (1981) who state: 'When the behaviour expected of an individual is inconsistent and there is ambiguity and conflict, the individual will experience stress, become dissatisfied, and perform less effectively' (Reprinted from *Social Science and Medicine*, **15**, 639–47, 1981, with kind permission from Pergamon Press Ltd., Headington Hill Hall, Oxford OX3 0BW, UK.) No attempt was made to measure the level of stress objectively; only the descriptive, subjective terminology used by nurses to describe their stress was recorded. The terms 'very stressful' and 'extremely stressful' were used by nurses to describe their stress levels. A 'very stressful' role was qualified as one where stress was continuous, which made heavy demands on the nurse emotionally, physically and socially, and where action in the form of explicit, intentional support, advice and help was needed. An 'extremely stressful' role was perceived by nurses to indicate 'unrelenting' stress, making it 'virtually impossible to care for patients and to do one's job efficiently'.

As well as the use of these terms, words such as 'pressure', 'concern', 'worry' and 'frustration' were also used by nurses in response to questions on their role; the use of these descriptive words indicated additional, smouldering levels of stress which nurses, on further questioning, confirmed.

What was the extent of nurses' stress? Of the 21 ward sisters interviewed, many (71%, $n = 15$) stated their role had a 'high' level of stress; some (24%, $n = 5$) said their role was 'very stressful'; and one (5%, $n = 1$) said her role had 'great stress'.

The majority of staff nurses (90%, $n = 67$) acknowledged a tolerable, though unacceptable, level of stress; the remaining 10% ($n = 7$) did not acknowledge any stress in their role.

ACKNOWLEDGED CAUSES OF STRESS

The common causes of stress identified by ward sisters included those of inadequate staffing levels, especially the mix of skills, inordinate workload (clinically and administratively), trying to maintain proper standards and quality of care and having little or no time to talk to and be with patients and care for them as they would wish.

Staff nurses generally echoed these causes as a source of stress in their role but, in addition, included those of constantly having to borrow equipment due to the lack of sufficient hoists, syringes and dressings, defective equipment, e.g. broken sphygmomanometers, coping with doctors' ward rounds (especially identified by recently registered nurses), lack of support in their job together with lack of guidance and counselling, relating to their professional and social problems and having to come to terms with their new responsibilities on qualifying and on appointment to their first post.

Many (80%) staff nurses emphasized the lack of proper preparation for their job, particularly emphasizing the lack of reality and inappropriateness of their preparation for meeting the needs and the demands of their job. Many said they were flung in at the deep end and left unsupported, and had to find their own solutions to the many complex problems associated with their role.

How did other professionals see nurses' stress? Unit nurse managers perceived little if any detectable (not more than expected of staff working in a stressful environment) stress associated with their role.

In contrast, senior nurse managers perceived much stress in the nurses' role, particularly for staff nurses, who they perceived especially as lacking the requisite authority, autonomy and necessary support and advice to do their job. There is a paradox here insofar as when nurse managers were questioned specifically on the extent of nurses' authority and autonomy, their responses were, to say the least, ambiguous and enigmatic. For example, they said nurses had the requisite authority and autonomy, but failed to use it; on the other hand, their responses identified their control over the power and freedom of the nurse to act. However, they now related this to one of the main causes of nurses' stress. They acknowledged the nurses' role to be particularly stressful, stating that it contained more stress than would normally be expected or tolerated, which they attributed to the shortage of resources, the nature and demands of ward practices and ward management and nurses attempting, in this climate, to meet demands additional to their expected role, for example requirements of the English National Board, e.g. those of supervising and teaching nursing students, for which they were not prepared. They further stated that the inadequate staffing of some wards, the lack of freedom for nurses to do their job and, most importantly, a lack of time for them to do their job properly contributed immeasurably to nurses' stress.

Many (88%) doctors, especially consultants, said nurses' stress resulted from the many constraints of their job, including 'nurses' limited authority and autonomy, too many bosses, demanding and wide-ranging responsibilities, lack of appropriate education and training and, more importantly, the inadequacy of their relevant expertise and experience to meet the demands of their role'. Many (70%) doctors indicated a lack of support and little appreciation by nurse management, and some doctors, of the real demands of their job.

Identified sources, frequency and intensity of stress as perceived by nurses

The terminology relating to the frequency and the intensity of stress is based upon the subjective, descriptive terms used by nurses. No attempt was made objectively to measure nurses' stress, because stress was not included within the terms of reference of the initial study. However, the problems of nurses' stress constantly recurred in the course of interviews (especially in the pre-pilot study) to the extent that the author felt it was too important to leave out of the study entirely and felt that it was such an important issue that it also warranted further, full investigation in a separate study.

COMMENT

From the foregoing analysis it is clear that events which predispose to stress are many and include the nature of the nurses' role, its elements, complexity and demands. Workload together with the many interpersonal relationships, lack of professional preparation and appropriate on-going development to meet the demands of their role were contributory factors. Currently nurses are affected by the additional stress of job insecurity, e.g. short-term contracts and job losses by closure of beds, units and hospitals.

The delivery of care places heavy demands on the nurse and requires the enactment of many roles, for which many nurses are not adequately prepared, e.g. nurse, manager, facilitator, mentor, communicator, counsellor, leader, etc., all of which are embodied in and required by the acknowledged role of ward sister and/or staff nurse.

Nurses hold expectations for their own role performance, i.e. their intention is to provide a service to their patients at a professional level, in keeping with their training and their responsibilities. If these expectations are not met, role conflict and role strain may lead to role stress, because of tension, frustration and anxiety which occur in their wake. Role stress thus exemplified – the causes, frequency and intensity which are outlined in Table 8.1 – are many and disabling, limiting nurses' job satisfaction by preventing them from ensuring the proper care and safety of their patients. Further stress is caused by potential censure from their employer and nursing statutory body for failing to meet their obligations.

Nurses' concerns were readily stated and included 'I get anxious about the pressure on staff but can't do anything about it. It is an added cause for concern when attempting to ensure the safety of patients. I constantly worry even at home after a busy day wondering if I have done everything properly. Nurses worry about the introduction of sophisticated technology they are expected to use after the minimum period of training and the level of decisions they have to make without support'. These current concerns of nurses were identified in the Briggs report (Briggs, 1972) two decades ago and remain unaddressed. Briggs found 'The changing nature of medical care has added to the strain imposed on nursing and midwifery staff – anxiety about errors in medical dosage, fears of machinery, ethical problems, and uncertainty over rapid decisions to be made in a time of crisis' (para. 581, p. 176). The findings of this report in relation to nurses' stress are supported by many other works before and after its publication, including those of Benne and Bennis (1959), Revans (1964), Hingley et al. (1984), the Audit Commission (1991) and Seccombe and Ball (1992).

HOW DID NURSES COPE WITH THEIR STRESS?

What action was taken locally, at district level, to enable nurses to cope with their stress? What provision was made to deal with nurses' stress nationally? What priority was given to the acknowledgement/prevention of nurses' stress by nurse managers? By the profession?

In the 20 wards studied, only one ward sister provided an informal system within the ward in an attempt to help nurses cope with their stress, insofar as it affected and was related to the ward. This system entailed a nurse choosing a colleague anonymously from the ward team to be her counsellor. In practice, a staff nurse or an enrolled nurse would choose another staff nurse or enrolled nurse. The ward sister, not having a counterpart on the ward, had to find another person, usually another ward sister external to her ward, to discuss her problems. On questioning the usefulness of this approach, the ward sister said 'It works very well in the absence of other support, though it has some shortcomings, e.g. limited time and the lack of expertise as "nurse counsellor", a role we undertake without any training'.

There were no appointed persons as counsellors, accredited or otherwise, or official systems within the districts and hospitals studied to deal with staff stress. Despite most managers being aware of its existence, their responses showed that they felt it was not a major concern, with unit nurse managers stating 'There is little appreciable detectable stress in nurses' role', and senior nurse managers acknowledging nurses' stress by stating 'Stress is caused by nurses' extended role; doctors want nurses to do a lot of things they don't want to do themselves, e.g. taking i.v. samples, giving i.v. injections, intubating patients and doing ECG'.

At the national level, the counselling service provided by the Royal College of Nursing, 'Counselling Help and Advice Together' (CHAT), employs two full-time counsellors and three part-time counsellors. (According to the evidence given in a UKCC (1987) report, the NHS nursing workforce in the UK consisted, in 1985, of 509 000 whole-time equivalents.) Counselling surgeries are mainly held in London and, according to the Royal College of Nursing, are fully booked, especially since the 'regrading' of nurses was introduced. However, counsellors, on request, visit centres outside London for a period of two days monthly.

In 1989, because of demand, a national, voluntary association was set up, namely the National Association for Staff Support (NASS) (Owen, 1989), within the health care services. The association consists of professionals with a common interest in the co-ordination and development of staff support resources within the health care services. The aims of the association are 'to identify and promote good staff support practices within the health care services' and 'to establish and maintain a national network of those concerned with promoting staff support'.

In addition to these services, the Nurses' Welfare Service, which is based in

London, has over the past seventeen years provided 'crisis intervention' for nurses, midwives and health visitors faced with the prospect of having their names removed from the professional nurses' register. The service gets financial support from different agencies, including the Royal College of Nursing and the United Kingdom Central Council for Nursing, Midwifery and Health Visiting.

The service offers information and advice when a nurse's professional conduct or fitness to practice is to be investigated; help, if appropriate, in preparing statements for the investigating committee; further support if the nurse is referred to one of the professional conduct committees of the UKCC; and continued counselling to enable the nurse to identify and work through the problems which have led to the crisis. On discussion of the situation with the person in charge, it was stated that 'many nurses referred for counselling were alleged to be "drug dependent" and/or "alcohol dependent"'.

In the light of the obvious lack of support and advice facilities, especially locally at district and regional level, how did nurses cope with their stress? What did they do? Many nurses indicated their unease at the official lack of acknowledgement together with the lack of resources/facilities available to them to enable them cope with their problems and stress at regional and district levels. They felt that some person or system should be made available within the hospital, to enable them to discuss their problems and worries. On discussion it became apparent that many nurses, especially staff nurses, were making 'a cry for help' before it was too late, i.e. before becoming ill and/or involved in more serious situations, in the hope of obtaining help and support for their problems.

The situation outlined by nurses and the concern shown by them indicates an urgency in coping with this socially and emotionally disabling problem, in the interest of themselves, their colleagues, patients and the professional and economic integrity of the service as a whole. The mechanisms described by nurses to help them to cope with their stress were, at best, temporary measures and included 'talking with family and friends, have a drink, have a good cry and when things get really bad, take a few days off'.

It is difficult in a retrospective study of nurses' absenteeism, attrition rates and sickness to identify stress-related causes. However, in response to the many nurses who indicated appreciable levels of stress in their job, a request was made to senior nursing managers of both district health authorities for information on the attrition, sickness and absentee rates of ward sisters, staff nurses, enrolled nurses and senior (third year) nursing students during the previous five years, in an effort to discover any link between these and the perceived levels of nurses' stress, i.e. medical certification of stress, anxiety, exhaustion, etc.

Nursing students and enrolled nurses were included because of the evidence presented, which underlined their inordinate workload and responsibilities and their lack of supernumerary status.

Senior nurse managers agreed to provide the information requested. However, neither district was able to provide information for the requested five-year period, as 'records were officially kept only during the past two years'. Subsequently, because of a stated 'computer failure', district health authority 2 was unable to supply the information requested. However, a nursing officer with responsibility for maintaining such data said 'the attrition rates, sickness and absenteeism of staff were not significant, and did not reflect any undue problem'.

A summary of the analysis on absenteeism, with the use of the chi-squared test, based on the information supplied by district health authority 1, is as follows: For a period of six months on the medical unit, sisters (whole-time equivalents (WTE), 8) had absences of 9 days, staff nurses (WTE, 30) had absences of 136 days and enrolled nurses (WTE, 11) had absences of 112 days. This gives an average absence over six months of 5.24 days. For a similar period on the surgical unit, sisters (WTE, 17) had absences of 62 days, staff nurses (WTE, 53) had absences of 193 days and enrolled nurses (WTE, 26) had absences of 143 days. This gives an average over six months of 4.15 days. The differences, taking both units together, between enrolled nurses and staff nurses and ward sisters is quite significant. In this respect, 108 sisters and staff nurses lost 400 days; 37 enrolled nurses lost 255 days.

Marked differences were indicated. In the medical unit, 11 enrolled nurses lost 112 days or over 10 days each, and in the surgical unit, 26 enrolled nurses lost 143 days, or 5.5 days each. Nursing students (intake 67) had a total of 581 days' sickness over a period of two years, or 8.67 days each.

These findings are both significant and interesting in the context of nurses' absenteeism, though regrettably, in the absence of factual information on the underlying individual causes for the absenteeism, nurses' stress as a causative factor can only be conjecture on the basis of information supplied by nurses themselves, which may be incomplete.

However, despite the absence of statistical evidence, it is important to note that on surgical wards, which had staff numbers (WTEs) greatly in excess of medical wards, the absentee rate was greater.

Some clues as to the causes underlying these differences may reside in the different profile of medical and surgical wards. For example, on medical wards patient dependency was agreed by nurses, nurse managers and doctors to be 'high' (above average). On surgical wards patient dependency was agreed to fluctuate between 'high' and 'intermediate' (average care). In addition the average stay of patients on medical wards was 14 days; this differed substantially from the average stay in surgical wards, which was six days.

In the study, the perceptions of nurses, nurse managers and doctors of the ethos of the clinical environment showed marked differences between medical and surgical wards. In this respect, surgical wards were perceived to be 'ordered', 'stable' and 'predictable' insofar as the admission of patients in the main was regular and predictable, i.e. mainly arranged, predetermined admissions. Also, surgical operations with few exceptions were predetermined. The nursing and medical regimes were precise and unequivocal; the discharge of patients was orderly. Despite this regularity and predictability of operation and care, many nurses agreed there was an 'additional' workload because of the rapid turnover of patients. Also, and more importantly, many nurses, ward sisters and staff nurses said their level of job satisfaction was greatly reduced by this as well as by the frequent practice, because of a limited number of beds, of transfer of patients to other wards, sometimes to medical wards, before their discharge, in an effort to secure beds for other 'arranged' and some emergency admissions. This added to their frustration of not seeing the patient get well and go home, which had an immeasurable destructive effect on their job satisfaction.

Medical ward staff perceived less 'stability' and 'orderliness' in their environment, as well as a degree of 'disruptiveness' and 'unpredictability' and the additional stress of coping with patients who had attempted suicide and those suffering from mental deterioration. During periods of observed behaviour these findings were evident. An attempt was made to relate the absenteeism rates locally with national rates, but no figures were available from the RCN, DSS, or UKCC for discrete specialities to enable the comparison.

The fact that little is done to control, regulate and reduce/alleviate stress in nurses is an indictment of the profession which refuses to acknowledge the potentially serious, damaging and ultimately disabling effects of stress on nurses themselves, their patients, the nursing profession, and the National Health Service as a whole.

The cost to the service, although largely 'hidden', in the disruption of the nurse, the patient and the organization, in terms of human misery and debilitation, is potentially great. It is therefore incumbent on nurse managers in conjunction with nursing statutory and professional bodies to anticipate nurses' professional/clinical problems; to regulate nurses' workload so that, at a given time, the workload is appropriate to their skills, knowledge and expertise; to ensure proper support and counselling as regular and ongoing essentials of nurses' professional development; to make clear the boundaries of the nurses' role; and to ensure that nurses' aspirations and job satisfaction are met as fully as possible. In this context, it is incumbent on them seriously and as a matter of urgency to regulate the glaring gap between nurses' principal aspiration, their desire to nurse and care for patients, which many perceive to be the primary focus of their role, and their education, training and development. To correct the situation, the management of stress should include identifying, preventing and/or correcting the many causes of stress. This includes addressing issues of manpower and, in this context, approaching in a positive manner the interviewing, selection, induction, education and training of staff which are vital prerequisites to sound nurse performance, together with examining and defining the nurses' role. Factors which negate job satisfaction, e.g. poor working conditions, lack of status, inadequate salary, inappropriate or inadequate training, lack of support and diminished career prospects must be corrected.

POSITIVE ACTION

The nursing professional and statutory bodies together with the employing authorities should use the current mode of major change as a catalyst to be more realistic in terms of the needs and demands of nurses, more personalized and more humanized. The new educational and organizational initiatives should embody, at the commencement of studentship, a support/counselling system which should have parity of quality nationally and continue throughout the nurses' career; be always available and accessible at the point of need; be properly resourced and not reliant on the well-intentioned but inadequate service available at present.

The difficulties in setting up a service of this nature are many with the most important aspect being the vehicle to choose to inaugurate such a service. I would propose that the Nurse Executive Director postholders undertake such an initiative as a matter of urgency. They are ideally placed to undertake such a task, as they should understand the problems, stress and anxiety nurses encounter; should be able to envisage what type of support they would have benefited from during their own career; could use the network of fellow postholders to organize a national forum which in turn should give them a greater say, a louder voice in presenting the initiative to their own boards as well as to the Department of Health.

Stress and anxiety prevention and/or alleviation methods should be developed. In this respect Bowman (1986) advises:

> A more comprehensive and positive approach to the education of nurses to inform them of the problems relating to stress should be undertaken as well as adopting a more positive psychological vetting of nurses on selection in an effort to screen and advise those potentially prone to stress and anxiety, perhaps using personality assessment tests, many of which are available, including Cattell's 16PF Questionnaire [Cattell and Ebel, 1964] and Eysenck Personality Inventory [Eysenck, 1963] ... Management primarily must ensure the proper resourcing of jobs. It must also monitor staff to detect any unacceptable level of stress. In addition, it must support staff by all means available, i.e. be ensuring their proper induction, training and development, avoiding undue work demands, and ensuring adequate resources, and by counselling them when necessary. Most importantly, management must use the potential of their staff, their skills, knowledge and expertise, thus increasing their job satisfaction, security, performance and enabling their self-actualisation.

(Paras 1/3, pp. 184/5)

Nurse managers must monitor the environment in which nurses work and for which they are accountable (UKCC, 1992). Professional and statutory bodies together with management must ensure that the nurses' role, in terms of its responsibility, authority, accountability and autonomy, is realistic, appropriate to the demands of the job and receives appropriate recognition, by ensuring the education of nurses to meet its demands; together with affording role occupants appropriate status and conditions of service with the possibility of including assertiveness training in the curriculum in order that nurses have their own responsibility in ensuring their own authority and autonomy. The role of management should be to ensure that they do everything possible to prevent stress occurring, by regulating the environment in which nurses work. However, management must also provide resources and facilities to enable nurses to cope with their stress if it occurs. Of equal importance is the part played by individual nurses, who must discuss and share problems and support their colleagues (UKCC, 1992; paras 4, 6 and 14). Above all, they must develop coping behaviours – skills to enable them to cope with their stress.

PARALLELS WITH OTHER PROFESSIONS

In this stress unique to the nursing profession? To answer this question an attempt was made by the author in the interest of further clarification and comparison to obtain information on stress in other professions. Letters were sent to some professional organizations inviting the following information.

- information on known, acknowledged stress (statistics);
- known causes of stress;
- number (if any) of counsellors (accredited or other);
- counselling support services available to staff.

Approaches to professions, including local authority, insurance, police and clergy (Roman Catholic), met with a limited response: whilst they recognized that staff suffered stress-related problems, they had not researched or done anything constructive about monitoring or evaluating it.

For example, during discussion with a senior officer of a local authority, it was stated that staff experienced an appreciable level of stress, and it was especially emphasized that young employees were substantially affected. No method of preventing, assessing, recording or managing stress was used. Counsellors were not employed. The officer added that following seven weeks on sick leave, staff were seen by the occupational health nurse and, if deemed necessary by her, were referred to the visiting GP and/or an appropriate voluntary organization; there was no follow-up.

The policy as outlined is incomplete, as there was no means of identifying stress at the early stages and affecting the individual and appeared only to be acted upon when it became a problem to the employer, i.e. when the employee took time off. This situation was further aggravated if the inadequate referral system was not monitored or evaluated.

A spokesperson for the Roman Catholic Church at national level said: 'I fear the lack of time does not allow me to get down to any research. Even though there is a treatment/rehabilitation centre in operation, for marked cases of stress, no figures are kept. There is no proper facility at diocesan and/or parish level for the diagnosis, monitoring or evaluation of stress; there are no formal counselling services available though many diocese have organized their own informal systems. We have no accredited counsellors'.

A response from the Occupational Health Psychologist responsible for support facilities for the Fire and Police Services said: 'We have inadequate information on fire and police officer stress and as [I am] a part-time employee lack of time prevented collation of information'. However, informal discussion with police and fire officers revealed an appreciable level of stress, mainly due to demands of the job, including change, workload (mainly administrative), dealing with people at large, lack of training in interpersonal skills, lack of authority to make basic decisions relating to work, lack of support, no-one to confide in, due, rightly in our opinion, to restrictions of rules of confidentiality and unsocial working hours, which adversely affected social and family life.

The response to the request for information from the Association of British Insurers stated: 'ABI has not yet undertaken research into the possible effects of occupational stress either within the insurance industry or the insured working population, largely because it is unlikely that any employer will be prosecuted under current health and safety legislation for any risk to health which an employee claims he has suffered as a result of stress'. In contrast to the above policy, it is interesting to note that Guide Dogs for the Blind Association (1993) have commissioned research into the prevention, causes and effects of stress in guide dogs. The Association saw this as important, stating

We needed to evaluate stress in guide dogs because we are very aware that if this is ignored vulnerable blind people are put at risk. We also have put into operation, staff profiling at interview before being employed by GDBA, monitoring of stress, evaluation of our support counselling systems; we do employ occupational psychologists and accredited counsellors. We feel this is not only a desirable but a vital part of human resource management because of the responsibility we have for the safety, rehabilitation and training of blind people and our staff deserve the best support we can offer them.

Nurses

In contrast to the latter organization nurses, who work in a naturally stressful environment, described by Revans (1964) as 'an organism characterised by anxiety' (para. 2, p. 91), have very little support. In this respect, following a general enquiry regarding stress in nursing to the Chief Nursing Officer of the Department of Health, it was stated:

> The Department does not collect detailed information on stress within professional groups; but one department supports the provision of counselling and support services for staff, as good practice. Decisions concerning their provision are a matter for local management. The number of BAC accredited counsellors employed in support services for staff is not collected centrally.

The Chief Nursing Officer advised that I contact the NASS, RCN and the Health and Safety Executive to obtain the information requested.

The General Secretary of the National Association for Staff Support in the Health Care Services (NASS) stated: 'I regret there is no accurate information available on several of your requests such as known causes and support services . . . Apply to the Department of Health for information on counselling services'.

The Royal College of Nursing (CHAT) (RCN, 1993) has on its staff 2.5 counsellors, all of whom hold a Diploma in Counselling Skills, one of whom is BAC accredited. The counselling service serves a population of some 500 000 nurses. The total number registered with the counselling service, January 1992–June 1992, was 1117; the number of counselling/advice sessions was 1724. The total number of nurses registered for counselling during the period July 1992–December 1992 was 513; the number of counselling/advice sessions was 1169.

In the latter period the age span of clients was 18–63 years; the main category of nurse for counselling was UKCC registered nurse (82%); the main regions for client counselling were NW Thames (26%), NE Thames (19%) and SE Thames (14%).

The main categories of problem for counselling were relationships (28%), emotional problems (26%), work-related stress (16%) and illness (7%). The ethnic origin of clients for counselling was substantially (86%) White European.

It is evident from the foregoing information that a counselling services is needed. It could be argued that a few thousand counselling sessions in comparison to the 500 000 workforce does present a major problem. Clearly, the CHAT figures cannot reflect the extent of the problem as it is under-resourced, e.g. there are 2.5 counsellors to cover a large demographically scattered population of nurses of differing grades and responsibilities; the surgeries are always full and they are only able to offer a limited service to clients because of time, staffing and travel to the regions every three months.

Other sources from which information on occupational stress was obtained included the medical profession, MIND (National Association for Mental Health) and the Health and Safety Executive (Technology Division).

The BMA in a recent publication (1992) are concerned that 'Stress is a largely hidden problem in the profession with very few statistics available to demonstrate its true extent' (para. 2, p. 1). This publication, while acknowledging that information on hospital doctors was anecdotal, identified elements deemed to be particularly stressful. These included the undermining of the role of clinicians by managers, e.g. in prioritizing patient lists; the requirement for clinicians to take on a managerial role; increased paperwork, much of which is felt to be unnecessary; and lack of proper consultation.

Stressors of GPs were identified to include the new phenomenon of business stress, the imposition of indicated prescribing amounts, the increased workload, restraints of the extracontractual referrals when the GP wanted the best for the patient, and redefined roles within the practice.

The publication, when discussing strategies for the reduction and management of stress within the profession, identified as a prerequisite 'recognition of its existence by the individual, by the representing profession, and those in health service management and government' (para. 3, p. 58). It acknowledged certain pressures which are avoidable and can be removed by good management and working practice as well as identifying specific areas where action can be taken to minimize stress. In this context, it is recommended that there be a restructuring and improving of medical education, including postgraduate training, and in this respect there should be increased flexibility in the career structure, use of sabbaticals, changes from full to part-time work and vice versa, and clarification of role, with increased emphasis on practical skills training for medical students and preregistration house officers. In addition, junior doctors' hours of work should be tailored to meet their needs and the needs of the health service; counselling and careers advice should be available to all doctors including the provision of fulltime medically qualified student counsellors to support students where necessary, as well as the provision of a counselling service in hospital, independent of the doctor's firm, who have the ability to refer doctors on to more specific therapists.

Finally, the publication advised a need for a fundamental view of the working relations between the different groups in the care services; management training should become an essential part of undergraduate and specialist training; the provision of an occupational health service, because 'It is ironic that health facilities for the medical profession are frequently inadequate' (para. 3, p. 73).

The foregoing strategies could readily be adopted by the nursing profession, as many of the identified problems and anomalies are indentical to those encountered by nurses. In the light of potential and/or actual divisions between practice nurses, doctors and managers, it would be advisable to look at stress collectively and agree appropriate and meaningful strategies by tripartite participation and consultation in an effort to establish an overall beneficial effect to the service, staff and patients.

A recent study by Dr Donald Currie (1992) includes the sampling of a total of 15 000 staff by use of postal questionnaires sent to four NHS hospital trusts in south-central England which had a response rate of 42.4%. The findings of the study identified the following stressors common to all staff: poor communication, workload, staff shortage, leadership (often described as 'over-authoritarian') and poor management style, i e distancing between staff and management, described as 'ivory tower syndrome'.

The main coping mechanisms identified by staff included 'smoking and drinking'.

Finally, 80% of respondents said they suffered work stress; 36% were receiving treatment. Clearly, these findings need to be treated seriously and addressed as a matter of urgency by the profession, managers, and health services.

The MIND survey

The MIND survey (1992) included sampling of 109 companies. Stress was defined as 'a symptom or manifestation of personal or work problems'.

The recession, leading to fears of redundancy and pressure to perform, was considered to be the main factor contributing to stress in companies. This was not evaluated on an individual employee basis but was based on company information.

Nearly one-third of southern-based companies (30%) said the recession had increased stress levels by 'more than average', compared to 21% in the north, with the biggest contributing factors to stress being pressure to perform, fear of redundancy/job uncertainty, recession, change or the pace of change, personal or home life, and increased job load due to the reduction of staff. Half of the 109 companies in the survey (50%) believed that moodiness could be caused by stress, while 63% said that stress manifested itself as a headache or migraine.

Larger companies showed a greater understanding of stress: 78% of businesses with over 10 000 employees recognized that a headache or migraine could be caused by stress, while only one-third of companies with under 49 staff did.

What the survey demonstrated was the damaging effects of stress on staff performance, with 21% of companies estimating that 25–50% of all absenteeism from work was attributable to stress and a further 27% estimating that 10–25% of absenteeism was similarly attributable. The authors concluded 'stress is evidently a problem that is increasing'.

It is suggested that the way forward lies in the willingness of companies, both large and small, to recognize and deal with stress. Larger companies put greater emphasis on dealing with stress and tended to offer professional counselling, compared with small companies, which only offered time off to 'sort things out'. In this context, staff may be referred for internal professional counselling, referred for external professional counselling, referred to welfare/health resources within company and/or monitored by the human resources director.

Health and Safety Executive

A paper by Sykes (1988) for the Health and Safety Executive identified 'sick building syndrome'. Sick building syndrome is defined as 'a building in which complaints of ill-health are more common than might reasonably be expected' (Finnegan et al., 1984).

The paper is detailed and contains much useful information on working environment, lighting, VDUs, dissatisfaction and psychological causes, including 'frustration at lack of environmental control, poor management and discomfort'. The paper reviewed published information on 'sick building syndrome', the cause of the reputedly high incidence of sickness amongst occupants of sealed, mechanically ventilated buildings. It discussed symptoms, common features of 'sick buildings' and possible causes and stated on the basis of reported cases that there appears to be no single cause but a series of contributing factors' (Summary, p. i).

Symptoms and prevalence were summarized by the WHO (1982) as eye, nose and throat irritation, sensations of dry mucous membranes and skin, erythema (skin rash), mental fatigue, headaches, high frequency of airway infections, cough, hoarseness, wheezing, itching and unspecified hypersensitivity, nausea and dizziness. Possible causes of sick building syndrome included:

- airborne pollutants, e.g. chemical pollutants from the building occupants, fabric and furnishings, office machinery and from outside; airborne dust and fibres; microbiological contaminants from carpets, furnishings, building occupants or from the ventilation or air conditioning system;
- odours;
- lack of small negatively charged ions in the air;
- inadequate ventilation/fresh air supply;
- low relative humidity;
- poor working environment or discomfort due to high temperatures, inadequate air movements, stuffiness and poor lighting;
- general dissatisfaction or psychosomatic causes.

The paper stated that 'Many of these are interrelated subjects and "sick building syndrome" may well result from the simultaneous effect of a number of challenges' (para. 2, p. 3). Many of the identified causes could realistically be related to the environment in which many nurses work, particularly those of building design, lighting, heating and poor ventilation.

The Whitehall Study

Marmot *et al.* (1991) studied 10 314 civil servants – 6900 men and 3414 women – and investigated the social gradient in morbidity of British civil servants. The survey had as its target population all men and women aged 35–45 working in the London offices of twenty civil service departments. The authors stated:

> Our findings show that socio-economic differences in health status have persisted over the twenty years separating two Whitehall studies (the first study began in 1967). In social class difference in morbidity we found an increased association between employment grade and prevalence of angina, electrocardiogram evidence of ischaemia and symptoms of chronic bronchitis. Self-perceived health status and symptoms were worse in subjects of lower status jobs ... Jobs characterised by low control, low opportunity to learn and develop skills, and high psychological workload, are associated with increased risk of cardio-vascular disease from the contributory factor of these identified stressors ... attention should be paid to the social environment, job design and the consequences of income inequality in an effort to reduce morbidity and mortality rates.

This advice should be heeded and acted upon by the health services with particular regard to job design and educational development.

A survey on occupational stress on teachers in the UK (Travers and Cooper, 1992), in which questionnaires were sent to a random sample of 5000 teachers drawn from a cross section of school types, sector and teacher grades, revealed from a response of 1790 (36%) 'that in comparison to other highly stressed occupational groups, e.g. tax officers, GPs, dentists and nurses, teachers were experiencing significantly lower levels of job satisfaction than these other groups, and suffering from significantly higher levels of mental ill-health'.

Teachers were on average showing dissatisfaction with 'the opportunity to use their abilities; their hours of work; their physical working conditions; industrial relations between the management and teachers in their school; the recognition they get for good work; the way their schools are managed; and most dissatisfaction with the chances for promotion and most of all, their rate of pay'.

The authors found that on average teachers had 7 days absence (self-reported) in the last year; a total of 12 475 days were lost. Teachers believed that 57% of those days lost were due to stress-related causes. Twenty-three percent of the sample reported having a significant illness in the last year which was mainly related to stress, e.g. myalgic encephalomyelitis, stomach and bowel problems, asthma and chest problems, back and neck problems, and anxiety and depression'. In addition, 18.6% of the sample smoked, and of these, 8% believed their smoking was related to the relief of stress. Also, drinking appeared to be more stress-related, 21% saying their drinking was related to the relief of stress. In terms of drug-taking, 18% were prescribed drugs and of these 28% were taking antidepressants and 26% were taking sleeping pills.

Results revealed some sources of pressure (from 98 pressure items) including 'lack of support from Government; the constant changes taking place within the profession; the lack of information as to how changes were to be implemented; society's diminishing respect for the teaching profession; a salary that is out of proportion with workload; and the fact that a good teacher does not necessarily mean promotion'.

ANALYSIS

The professions identified, including nursing, and the evidence yielded indicate stressors which are common to these professions. Notable are those that relate to:

- the environment in which the person works, including its physical nature, such as heating, lighting and noise; workload; resources; the nature of authority and autonomy of the role occupant; and the nature and quality of working relationships;
- the person, including lack of recognition of one's worth to the profession/ organization; lack of status; lack of respect; lack of opportunity and encouragement to use one's skills, knowledge, initiative and creativity; lack of and/or stunted career prospects; inadequate or no development and updating; little or no involvement in decision making; poor industrial relations; and unsatisfactory conditions of service;
- management, including lack of overt acknowledgement of the existence of stressors and/or stress in its workers; absence of a stress prevention policy; lack of staff support and counselling service; lack of or inadequate staff development policy; no real recognition of staff commitment.

The cumulative effect of the identified inadequacies (not a complete catalogue) can lead to low staff morale, job dissatisfaction, staff disillusionment, absenteeism, sickness, worry, fear and in uncontrolled situations anxiety, stress and burnout. The causes of stress and the way staff in these studies coped with their stress, especially among the teachers studied, bore a close resemblance to what nurses said they did as a remedy for their stress, including smoking, drinking and drug taking.

From the evidence in this chapter it is clear that the nursing profession is not

unique insofar as its multiple pressures and often associated and acknowledged stress appear to be present in many other professions and jobs. Given
the present economic climate, nurses cannot and should not expect
preferential treatment. The NHS as a whole and local nurse management
cannot afford to ignore the existence of the levels of stress in the profession and
be constructive in its prevention, evaluation, monitoring and the provision of
support services, otherwise they do so at their peril!

The time is right to radically amend the anomalies that have blighted the
growth of the profession for so long. The ENB (1992) and UKCC (1986)
initiatives, together with the change to hospital trusts, could be used as a
catalyst to ensure quality assurance, not only to patients but also to nurses, in
their training, development and support.

Much literature is available evidencing nurses' stress, some of which has
already been identified in Chapter 3. In addition, the following are relevant:
Katz and Kahn (1978), Anderson (1973), Hardy and Conway (1978), Wieland
(1981), Gray-Toft and Anderson (1981), the Audit Commission (1991) and
Seccombe and Ball (1992).

There is an extensive bibliography on professional stress generally,
including Cooper and Marshall (1980), Cooper and Roden (1985), Cooper
and Watts (1987), Cooper, Rout and Faragher (1989), Khan and Cooper
(1990), Travers and Cooper (1991), Travers and Cooper (1992), Ostler and
Oon (1989) and Bunge (1989).

9	# Educational significance of findings: initiatives and proposals

PART ONE

BACKGROUND AND INITIATIVES

BACKGROUND

This chapter discusses initiatives within the NHS in general and nursing in particular, and their influence on the role of the professional nurse now and in the future. Proposals are made on the basis of main findings of the study together with an educational framework for their realization. The chapter is divided into two parts: Part one examines the background and initiatives and Part two discusses proposals and curriculum implications.

The practice of nursing, the professional nurse and the profession of nursing are at the crossroads; much change is contemplated in the realignment and the redirection of the nursing profession, to launch it successfully, constructively and effectively into the 21st century.

A superficial glance at the initiatives currently being addressed, including those of Project 2000 (UKCC, 1986), Framework for Continuing Education and Higher Award (ENB, 1992b, 1992c), *National Health Service and Community Care Act 1990* and NHS Trusts (DoH, 1989) evidences the envisaged changes will make great demands on nurses. If they are to be effective they will require a radical rethink and clearer definition of the nurses' role and a change in nurses' attitude and the attitude of the profession to the education of its nurses, especially regarding managerial and interpersonal skills as a prerequisite to ensuring a new direction.

It seems apropriate to quote the words of Professor Revans (1983) who aptly states:

> In any epoch of rapid change those organisations unable to adapt are soon in trouble, and adaptation is achieved only by learning, namely, by being able to do tomorrow that which might have been unnecessary today, or to be able to do today what was unnecessary last week. The organisation that continues to express only the ideas of the past is not learning, and training systems intending to develop our young may do little more than to make them proficient in yesterday's technique.
>
> *(Para. 1, p. 11)*

Over the years, to stem the decline of nursing, repeated attempts have been made by many notable reformers to change nursing education and practice. The investigations focused on the key areas of standards of care, education of nurses, communication and attrition rates for learners and registered nurses. These areas are clearly interrelated insofar as without the proper education, training and development of nurses, their skills, knowledge and ability to care for their patients are immeasurably curtailed.

The present study highlights some inadequacies based on the apparent ineptness and/or unwillingness of nurses and their profession to secure an acceptable standard of practice and make possible professional competence, confidence and integrity. Virtually all nurses interviewed perceived their basic training (pre-Project 2000, but the majority were trained 1–5 years prior to the study) as preparing them for a nursing/caring role and not a managerial/administrative role, which they were expected to undertake on qualifying.

Many (52%) ward sisters agreed that preparation for their role should start during the period acting as staff nurse, although some (33%) perceived development in the essential skills and knowledge of ward management to be ongoing. A few (14%) thought that training for their role should start on taking up their post.

Many (64%) staff nurses agreed that preparation for the managerial/administrative duties and the responsibilities of their role should start during the final year of their basic training. Some (32%) stated that the 'formal' (a preparatory course) preparation for their role should take place either on completion of their basic training or prior to registration. A few (4%) said that formal preparation should not be undertaken until they have completed at least one year in post.

When nurses were asked: Are nurses able to improve their professional competence, skills and knowledge? the majority said they could not do this 'completely' (ward sisters, 67%; staff nurses, 76%). For example, ward sisters said: 'You can make known to your nurse manager what you would like to do, but financial and staffing constraints, prevent. You can only go when staffing levels and workload, permit'. Staff nurses said: 'You have little control and influence over attending courses. You can request to go on a course, but are prevented because of workload and staff shortages. Nurse managers prevent nurses attending courses because they have no one to cover the ward'. This lack of development has not changed very much since the study was carried out. During discussions nurses and managers still maintain that they do not have the resources to ensure staff development. There seems to be an ongoing debate between nurse educationalists and nurse managers about the alleged imbalance in the allocation of resources for staff development. Managers complain that 'money is poured into student education for the development of new initiatives, even though these students could not be guaranteed work at the end of training, but we cannot get sufficient money for the development of essential skills and knowledge of registered nurses, who are in post'.

Some nurse educationalists counter this argument, stating:

> We don't disagree with the fact that postregistration staff development is underfunded. However, we do not accept the premise that you take funding from first-level training to correct the balance. There is a possibility that at the end of training students will not secure contracts but this is not a valid reason to impoverish the resourcing of their training. All you achieve with that philosophy is a badly trained first level of the profession, which will not only be damaging but will ultimately be economically unsound. Both pre- and postregistration training need to be properly resourced.

A report of the DoH Nursing Division (1989) echoes the concern of these managers: 'It must be a matter of concern that today's nurses do not routinely have facilities for periodic refreshment' (para. 2, p. 23). In a discussion with an officer of the RCN, it was stated 'an increasing number of nurses are not given contracts and the number of bank nurses is increasing even though no absolute figures are available on a national basis. Hospitals establish bank nursing in an attempt to secure a nucleus of nurses who have been trained by them for potential use'.

This scenario fails to deal with the central problem of nurses' contracts and brings in its wake additional problems and questions. How and when will these nurses obtain further training and development? Will they become disillusioned and seek alternative occupations? Will their basic training have been wasted at the cost to the taxpayer of approximately £45 000 per student? Sceptics will argue that other students of higher education courses are not guaranteed jobs. This is a fallow argument which should be condemned, as no organization, profession or country should waste the contribution a well-trained/educated workforce can make.

This waste of well-trained and skilled personnel belies the statement made by William Waldegrave (Foreword, Patient's Charter, DoH, 1991), 'The Government is also firmly committed to improving the Service – to creating a better National Health Service . . . [that] respects and values the immense resource of skill and dedication which is to be found amongst those who work for and with the National Health Service' (paras 4/8, p. 5). I am sure the large number of newly well-qualified nurses do not imagine that they enjoy the respect of Government when they are signing on the dole. Perhaps we are training too many nurses at a basic level and should redirect some of the resources to improving the skills of those already qualified, to meet current demands and responsibilities and more focused research into nurse manpower requirements.

On discussion with some nurse executive directors of NHS trusts, concern was also raised by them regarding nursing manpower: 'Manpower problems arise because of no rational planning at national level; finite resources dictate cost and quality of service. We are not good at manpower planning'.

The development of nurses into nurse managers, an inescapable role on qualifying now being adopted in NHS trusts, needs to be addressed seriously and urgently. Basic nursing qualifications coupled with a brief introduction to the philosophy and theory of management do not equip nurses to manage a complex service at ward level.

The philosophy of staff development, including nurse training, should be based on a thorough and effective system of selection, induction and appraisal with training objectives that meet the various needs of staff at a given period of their career. In the study there was little difference in the perceptions of nurses and other professionals in both districts and all clinical specialities of what they consider to be the best approach to the development of nurses in skills and knowledge, appropriate to the demands of their job.

The professional development of nurses after qualifying is unsatisfactory and a matter of concern, as evidenced in nurses' responses. For example, of the 21 ward sisters who took part in the study, four (20%) had not undertaken further training since qualifying (10–15 years before). The remaining 17 (80%) had only undertaken short courses of 2–7 days' duration. These were mainly on the skills of counselling, assessing and first-line management.

Of the 74 staff nurses interviewed, 32 (43%) had not undertaken further training; 25 (34%) had undertaken training lasting 0.5–2 days, mainly on matters relating to 'food hygiene'; 17 (23%) had received some training of 2–7 days' duration on the skills of assessing.

Many nurses interviewed had been qualified for several years, for example, 19 (26%) for 10–20 years and some more recently, 34 (46%) for 3–9 years.

The reasons frequently given by them for the absence of professional development included 'Lack of finance, lack of staff, no relief nurses and lack of career opportunity'. On being questioned about this gap, senior nurse managers said there was never enough money to ensure proper staff development and many staff were not interested because of family commitments or other reasons.

Professional education is an integral part of and a prerequisite for the understanding, implementation and success of the current educational and organizational initiatives. The skills perceived by nurses to enable the enactment of their roles as ward sister and staff nurse were almost identical. The perception of nurse managers and doctors on nurses' required skills supported these views (Tables 9.1, 9.2, 9.3 and 9.4).

INITIATIVES: CORRECTIVE APPROACHES?

The positive changes currently taking place in nursing within the framework of the EEC Nursing Directives (EEC, 1977, 1989), the *Nurses, Midwives and Health Visitors Act 1979,* Project 2000 and Framework for Continuing Education and Higher Award (ENB, 1992c) relating to nurses' education and development are sound and should go some way, in the context of other major organizational and educational initiatives, to correcting some longstanding and disabling anomalies.

Over the decades, nursing has created its own dilemmas by being closeted in its own predictability and lack of professional development. Standards have to be raised. In recent years the profession has become open to more public scrutiny and more accountable to that public for its actions and standards. Its predictability and security are gone. Accountability has to a degree always been present but, as expressed by executive nursing directors, it is now more explicit, insofar as senior managers are more conscious of litigation and risk than before. Initiatives include:

- *Caring for People: Community Care in the next Decade and Beyond* (DoH, 1989).
- *Working for Patients* (DoH, 1989). The proposals in both these Government White Papers were implemented in order to achieve an NHS that was highly efficient and good value for money through better management. These White Papers were the precursors of the following.
- *National Health Service and Community Care Act 1990*, which embraces the broad key objectives of promoting and developing services that enable people to live in their own homes wherever feasible and make provision for those who cannot. The key changes are that local authorities are more responsible, in collaboration with medical, nursing and other interests, for assessing individual need, designing care arrangements and securing their delivery.
- *The Patient's Charter* (DoH, 1991). The Charter is a central part of the Government's programme to improve and modernize the NHS and in this way ensure a service that meets the needs of patients and is responsive and accessible to the patient, setting and upholding the highest standards of care.
- Self-governing hospital trusts (DoH, 1989). It was envisaged that the formation of NHS Trusts would give patients more choice, produce a better quality service and encourage other hospitals to be even better, in order to compete.

Table 9.1 Skills and preferred specialist knowledge perceived by 21 ward sisters/charge nurses to enable them to do their job

Skills	Responses		Knowledge	Responses	
	n	%		n	%
Counselling (staff)	10	48	Clinical updating	15	71
Interpersonal (communicating and relating to others – staff, patients and relatives)	11	52	Applied psychology	6	29
Managerial (resources, human and non-human)	11	52	Research	4	19
Research	4	19			
Teaching	4	19	None	1	5

Table 9.2 Preferred educational methods perceived by 21 ward sisters/charge nurses to effect their educational development

Educational methods	Responses	
	n	%
Action learning	3	14
On-the-job training	8	38
Specialist short courses	9	43
Workshops	6	29

- The Nurse Executive Director post. Under the *NHS Community Care Act 1990*, provision was made that all Trusts that provide direct patient care must have among their executive directors a registered nurse or midwife.
- Project 2000 (UKCC 1986), intended as a wide-ranging review of educational preparation for nursing, midwifery and health visiting in the UK, advocating and concentrating on the background and nature of change envisaged.
- Framework for Continuing Professional Education and Higher Award (1992c). This is a major ENB initiative which provides a flexible system for continuing professional education.
- ENB Campus: Communication and Information (1992a). Established to enable those working in nursing, midwifery and health visiting education and practice to communicate and access important data bases more readily.

Table 9.3 Skills and preferred specialist knowledge perceived by 74 staff nurses to enable them to do their job

Skills	Responses		Knowledge	Responses	
	n	*%*		*n*	*%*
Communication (staff and patients)	21	28	Clinical updating and related research	39	53
Counselling (staff, patients and relatives)	58	78	Applied psychology	34	46
Interpersonal (relationships with others)	15	20			
Teaching	27	36			
Ward/staff management (planning, organizing, leading, motivating and supervising)	59	80			

Table 9.4 Preferred educational methods perceived by 74 staff nurses to effect their educational development

Educational methods	Responses	
	n	*%*
Action learning	13	18
On-the-job training	42	57
Specialist short courses	49	66
Workshops	13	18

These initiatives are an exciting challenge for the profession; a challenge that needs to be addressed and cannot afford to fail; a challenge that can only properly be addressed by a workforce that is well trained, highly motivated, secure and confident in their job and willing to accept major change. Many of these initiatives are ongoing but continue to encounter negative criticism. However, to ensure the full realization of their already stated objectives requires a concerted effort on the part of all those who are responsible for the delivery of care to the public and the satisfactory launch of nursing into the next century. Nurses form a substantial core of the workforce and as a direct result through their effective training, education and development will play a major part in the potential future success of these initiatives.

Caring for people

The document *Caring for People* (DoH, 1989) makes the following statements, all of which when enacted will substantially affect the role of the nurse, in the immediate future and beyond.

> All agencies and professions involved with the individual and his or her problems should be brought into the assessment procedure when necessary. These may include social workers, GP's, community nurses, hospital staff such as consultants in geriatric medicine, psychiatry, rehabilitation and other hospital specialities, nurses, physiotherapists, occupational therapists, speech therapists, community psychiatric nurses and others . . . The new assessment arrangement will involve significant changes in the way professional workers are expected to operate.
>
> *(Paras 3.2.5/3.2.13, pp. 19/20)*

The changes in *Caring for People* are intended to evolve a system whereby the interagency approach will enable the best possible use of resources and enable the individual to live in their own home or community if this is desired or praticable, by ensuring the best support services and life skills in order that they achieve their full potential.

The implication of these requirements and practices will affect the nature and operation of the nurses' role. The requirements are onerous! In the light of the findings on the nurses' role and nurses' stated inadequacies associated with their education, training and development together with their low morale, job insecurity and alleged subordination by other professionals, nurses need to be able to cope effectively and with confidence with these additional and potentially demanding responsibilities.

Areas that must be addressed with urgency, if nurses are to play a full part in this initiative, give rise to the following questions: Do nurses really know where accountability lies, with their new responsibilities under community care? For example, when the 'named' community care, ward staff nurse is arranging the discharge of a patient to their own home, they will have to do a lot more than automatically tick boxes on a discharge form, and instruct a patient to give the form to his/her GP. Will these 'named' nurses have to cope with this new and demanding role in addition to their heavy workload? Will nurses receive specialist training, e.g. Disability Awareness Training, to enable them to understand the needs of patients and work effectively with other agencies in the home environment, and create a realistic 'Care Plan' for the individual? Are health service personnel ready and able to take on this role? Will management continue to consider their staff to be effectively trained in this highly specialized area after superficial training lasting a few days or less?

It is interesting to note that the Guide Dogs for the Blind Association (GDBA) who, unlike the health services, do not have a statutory obligation to provide services, nevertheless prior to but in preparation for the enactment of the *NHS Community Care Act 1993* has taken very positive steps, by setting up a Training College (GDBA, 1993), that offers a ten-month, full-time residential course to train rehabilitation workers. The course aims to train existing and new GDBA personnel, as well as staff from local authorities and other agencies, in the very complex skills required to afford blind and partially sighted people the dignity and freedom to lead a supported, enhanced lifestyle within their own home and community, if they so wish. Caring for patients in the community continues to be linked, rightly or wrongly in some instances, with some anxiety as to whether the new service will prove to be effective in meeting patients' needs in a full and sensitive, humane way, always ensuring a quality service. Will there be the best use of resources, human and material, in the multiagency approach to care envisaged? Will the much discussed, cost effective, planned care materialize?

Change and the benefits of new legislation can only be achieved with a positive change of attitude coupled with the appropriate education and training of all staff. In addition, DHAs have a duty to secure the best service for their patients, be it from hospitals within the district over which they have control, from other districts, self-governing hospitals or from the private sector.

Working for patients

This White Paper (DoH, 1989) which followed Government review of the NHS aimed to ensure better health care of patients, a greater choice of services available and enhancement of job satisfaction of health care staff. To effect these aims the paper proposed making the service more responsive to the needs of patients, delegating more power and responsibility to the local level, establishing NHS Hospital Trusts; making available the necessary finance to hospitals that meet the needs of patients, reducing waiting times and adjusting the hours worked by junior doctors, improving GP services by enabling fund-holding practices, and delivering all health services on more business-like lines.

It is hoped that this will mean that it will be a better organized and managed service tailored to meet patient/community needs, satisfy staff aspirations and provide a quality service. Nurses must accept that services will be patient-led and they will have to change their attitude from a dogmatic, dictatorial delivery of service and learn the basic principles of customer care in a consumer demand situation by understanding the value of consumer participation and consultation in order to meet patients' needs effectively.

National Health Service and Community Care Act 1990

This Act embraces the main aims of the two previous White Papers. It contains a duty to consult organizations of users on the framing of community care plans and a specific duty to assess individual needs. Advisory circulars and consultation papers about the new Act from central government call for a clear separation between assessing need and meeting need. Better overall planning and a more rounded view of each person's needs seem to be the two principles at the heart of the new legislation.

The poor links between the hospital professionals, the local authority and the voluntary agencies has not been properly addressed in the Act and until they are addressed the objectives of the Act will be undermined.

The principles, philosophy and objectives of the Act are right, but there is a major problem in putting them into practice. Without the necessary structures and framework to enable implementation, especially within a reactive service, one that has often relied on crisis management, the effects and benefits of the Act will be rendered null and void.

The patient's charter

This charter (DoH, 1991) arises from the main principles of the *Citizen's Charter* by creating a better National Health Service, which will always put the patients first, provides services that meet national and local standards by participation and consultation with the user group, reflects people's views and needs and is responsive to them and values the immense resource of skill within the NHS.

The whole philosophy of the charter can be summarized as providing a highly efficient service achieved by better management as espoused in the two White Papers, *Working for Patients* and *Caring for People*. Charter rights are guaranteed. Can these rights realistically be guaranteed without the necessary framework in place in some neglected areas of the NHS? For example, the charter states: 'All health authorities should ensure that the services they arrange can be used by everyone, including children and people with special needs such as those with physical and mental disabilities' (para. 2, p. 13).

How will nurses meet the needs of people with sensory handicap? New statutes demand change. Improvement in services for people with a sensory handicap has been enshrined in legislation enacted in recent years, in particular, the *NHS and Community Care Act 1990*. This contains a duty to consult organizations of users on the framing of community care plans, a specific duty to assess individual need for social work services, rehabilitation and training.

The *Chronically Sick and Disabled Persons Act, 1970*, the *Chronically Sick and Disabled Persons (Amendment) Act 1976* and the *Disabled Persons (Services, Consultation and Representation) Act 1986* were important antecedents of this framework, more honoured in the breach than observance. Health and social services under the new Act will be required to assess each client's needs and develop a personal plan for that individual, ascertaining the client's own wishes. However, unless hospital staff are trained in disability awareness, they will be unable to assess the needs of the individual when developing a personal care plan.

The two main principles of this legislation are better planning and a total view of the needs of the individual. The new Act thus goes some way towards addressing the understated need, poor organization of services and people missing out on services. But putting the two principles into practice is inherently difficult for organizations concerned with people with a sensory handicap and their needs, because assessments are made within both the health authority and social services, and because the response to need has to come from several quarters.

Professionals often have an idiosyncratic attitude about the role and value of other agencies. Many professionals are unwilling to admit their lack of disability awareness, their lack of knowledge of services available and their lack of ability to identify the needs of the person being assessed.

There are some reservations on ethical issues and legitimate boundaries to passing medical or other confidential data on clients too readily from one agency to another. Heath authorities, social services and voluntary services have operated largely separately. There has been lip service paid to working together, but people have been sent or have passed from one sector to another. Each sector has its own perspective on the client, tackles part of the overall need, but does not seek to treat or advise, counsel or support the person as a whole. If services are to work together, these lacunae have to be addressed. The OPCS survey (1989) found that one in six of the population suffer one or more disabling/handicapping conditions. The majority of blind, partially sighted, deaf/blind, deaf and dysphagic people have additional health problems. Two-thirds of these groups will either have arthritis, a heart condition, hypertension, a physical infirmity or diabetes, to name but a few.

A high proportion of these clients (17% of hospital attenders, in- and outpatients) are people with a sensory handicap (RNIB, 1991), yet they encounter staff who cannot communicate with them, and fail to understand that it is the staff who have the communication problem and not the patient. Clients encounter staff who cannot advise them because they lack information and training in this area; cannot support or counsel them; cannot assess their needs, because they do not know what these needs are; and cannot hope to meet their needs. There is an urgent need for health authorities to look at the services they offer people with a sensory handicap. They will find the quality of service is abysmal. The rights and needs of this patient group have been totally ignored and must be dealt with.

Nurses will encounter practical problems when caring for the patient with sensory handicap. These are many and varied; central are the problems of communication, assessment and mobility. Nurse educators argue that the curriculum is already overloaded and can only include these important areas in a superficial way, but can they abrogate their responsibility in this way? Legislation states that they cannot. More importantly, nurses must be reminded of their accountability. For example, most nurses assume that they can write a communication to the prelingually deaf, but they do not realize the high degree of poor literacy skills of the deaf, and how inadequate and flawed this method is.

Currently if a prelingually deaf person attends a hospital, they have to be accompanied by a social worker or an interpreter. What happens to this patient's rights, especially those of confidentiality, freedom and dignity? How does the nurse know what is being signed to the client? Does the interpreter understand medical terminology and the implications or misinterpretation? Is the interpreter accountable for any inaccuracies, or is the nurse? These are questions that have not been addressed by health services and should be dealt with as a matter of urgency.

As a positive step forward the ENB should make sure that disability awareness training is an integral part of the curriculum, in order to begin to offer a quality service to one in six of the population. Health authorities and hospital trusts must ensure that the basic rights of patients with a sensory handicap are upheld, by employing communicators and ensuring that specialist skills of assessment are part of staff development. More importantly, they must be aware of the network of support agencies available to benefit the patient by formulating a directory of services. It is a time of change and this area is one that has been long overdue.

Self-governing hospital trusts

The Government's proposals for enabling hospitals and other NHS units and services to achieve self-governing status while remaining firmly within the NHS are set out in the White Paper *Working for Patients* (DoH, 1989). Among the many powers and responsibilities of each self-governing hospital vested formally in its NHS Hospital Trust will be: 'Determination of their own management structures without control from Districts, Regions or the NHS Management Executive', together with 'Determination of their own staffing structures and of the terms and conditions of service for staff' (para. 2.3, p. 3).

NHS Trusts would have powers to employ their own staff; but 'in general, the existing staff of a hospital would be likely to transfer from employment by their Health Authority to employment by the NHS Hospital Trusts', and 'DHAs in consultation with Shadow Trusts and the individuals concerned, will be responsible for identifying staff to be transferred' (paras 5.1/5.2, p. 25). The last statement begs many questions, especially on the continued employment of staff in post and most importantly their conditions of service, should they be transferred! On education and training: 'Trusts will be expected to play their part in training the staff they employ', and 'The size and complexity of nursing education and training, especially while Project 2000 is being introduced, will need careful consideration to ensure adequate standards and numbers are maintained' (paras 5.15/5.26, pp. 26/28).

The foregoing were some of the initial concerns raised about the launch of hospital trusts. Have things changed as we approach the fourth wave of hospital trusts? Discussions with the Department of Health on the progress of and the differences between trust and non-trust hospitals indicate that to date no formal evaluation has been undertaken 'on the before and after effects'.

An article by Kingman (1993) examines some of the issues since the introduction of the hospital as an NHS Trust. During an interview with the general manager, he stated 'In our first year we were beavering away to demonstrate the value of being a Trust. We had to show our efficiency and it was all much more gung-ho, breaking new ground as a trust (para. 2, p. 1465). The article found that disillusionment was setting in and people were voicing their frustration with it all. They felt they had 'knuckled down' the previous year, thinking that if they showed willing and treated more patients, their efforts would be rewarded by bigger budgets in the contracts for 1992/93. When contracts were initially set, it was found that they had to do the same amount of work without a corresponding increase in budget. The staff felt that during the first year there was a sense of pride insofar as their hospital, unlike others, did not close any beds. In addition staff felt an air of resignation as the Trust realized that there was nothing to gain by performing too well. They were also concerned about possible redundancies and the closure of one acute hospital in the district.

Two factors were bothering the staff and contributing to the pressure put on their hospital by the purchasers. First was 'the demand that the Freeman should deliver cash releasing cost improvements of 2%. In previous years cost improvements have been brought about to do, for example, 2% more work for the same amount of money. In 1993/94 the Freeman has been asked to do the same amount of work for 2% less'. The final word from the general manager was that 'The key to success is to satisfy the purchasers' demands. That is tough, but we will get there – we must'.

Inevitably, the setting up of NHS Trusts has had teething problems. The transition needs time for adjustment, time for people to change attitudes and time for people to acquire the necessary skills for their new roles and different emphasis. There are areas of impasse, as stated in the foregoing article, between the perceptions of the professional/clinical staff and the general manager. The professional staff perceive that because they are 'doing more they should be rewarded with an increase in resources', whereas the general manager is looking for 'more done for less', implying there is a need for greater efficiency. There is nothing basically wrong with this philosophy as long as quality assurance is built in and not sacrificed for quantity. A new opportunity for nurses to have a real voice in policy making and to motivate other grades has been brought about by the development of the nurse executive director post.

Nurse executive director

A report (DoH, 1992) gives a nursing perspective on the role and function of the nurse executive director post in first-wave NHS Trusts as 'an attempt to capture at the end of the first year of operation the views of nurse executive directors on their achievements in establishing a range of roles' (Foreword, para. 2, p. 1).

Data were collected using an in-depth personal interview and questionnaire with 24 nurse executive directors from first-wave trusts in 1992. The sample of 24 represented 12 of the 14 regions in England and a range of types of Trust organizations, including Acute Hospital Trusts, Acute Teaching Trusts, Whole District Trusts, Mental Health/Learning Disability Trusts, Community Trusts and Specialist Trusts. The core functions of the nurse executive director include ensuring that nursing services are organized to provide an effective delivery of nursing care to individuals and to provide leadership to nurses, midwives and health visitors through the development, implementation and evaluation of policies consistent with the goals and objectives of the Trusts.

The nature of the post in terms of role and function is as varied as the services offered by each individual Trust. However, they all have common elements which include:

- leadership of nursing practice;
- leadership of the profession;
- corporate leadership;
- direct/operational management;
- human resources management and quality assurance.

The role occupants are faced with a demanding task which from their comments most appear to be approaching with enthusiasm and a determined positiveness. 'With nurses making up the largest number of staff within the Trusts, sound leadership and promotion of nursing is essential'. 'My job is to look after and develop staff. Theirs is to deliver service'.

With regard to the changes in their post, only two respondents said their role had not changed. Those who said there had been change commented that their role had shifted from a nursing concentration to corporate issues, e.g. strategy and financial issues, or shifted from a focus on internal issues to external issues, e.g. liaison with purchasers and outside entities. When respondents were asked how they had changed one commented, 'Because we are in changing times, the only constraint is change. We must work more flexibly for current times but may need to turn the whole organization around to meet the future. It is important for nurses to concentrate on the visionary work beyond the strategic – not just the here and now'.

Respondents identified areas of skills and knowledge which they perceived would enable them to do their job more effectively and included 'Prioritizing and planning, policy analysis, problem solving, political and negotiating skills, people management, change management, managing across inter-organizational and inter-professional boundaries, marketing, contracting and financial management'.

To obtain further opinions from some nurse executive directors, to establish if another year had made any marked difference, some were written to and others were interviewed. The following are a random selection of comments from nurse executive directors in Acute Hospital Trusts during interview who felt there had been little or no change. 'The philosophy of staff management remains unchanged since before Trusts were set up'. 'Trusts have no influence on caring. Care is still being delivered in the same manner'. 'Drive for NHS Trusts is a political ideology. Nursing students are still not supernumerary. There is little real debate between provider and purchaser. Providers hold the main influence, the real power, they hold the purse strings. Each prepare a plan identifying priorities though ultimately the purchasing authority decide'. 'Manpower problems continue because there is no rational planning at national level. Finite resources dictate cost and quality of service'. 'There is a lot of stress at middle and senior manager levels largely due to explicit local accountability for the service'. 'Ward sisters now have less stress because they now have budgetary control and day-to-day responsibility of ward management'.

In contrast, others interviewed felt it was a time of much change. 'The philosophy of the role is one of close team approach, corporate identity, e.g. shaping of values in which we have major influence in the policy making. The provision of resources is more personal, can decide and see the results which leads to considerable job satisfaction by being in a position to influence nursing practice and development'. 'Accountability has always clearly been present though not litigation and risk conscious[ness] before'. 'Even though separate plans are prepared to establish priorities, i.e. provider/purchaser, there is usually good dialogue and in the event of an impasse, this is dealt with by the RHA and/or a Trust Outpost Body (monitoring role responsible to Management Executive)'. 'Manpower and other resources continue to present problems; we are not good at manpower planning. Most nurses on registration, if satisfactory, are offered permanent contracts; there is also an established nurse bank, though agency nurses are rarely employed'. 'Stress, different stressors are at work, one of which is accountability in developing a nursing service and ensuring proper staff development. Ward sisters have more responsibility and more freedom but also more accountability and resulting stress increase'. 'No problems encountered or perceived in the nurse/management chain of command'.

A nurse executive director of an NHS Acute Teaching Trust during interview said 'Role has evolved and embodies head of nursing. Role requires stamina and survival skills. The stressors of role are in part, due to the speed of change and uncertainty of outcome, because of the rationalization currently taking place in the NHS. There is concern regarding the potential effects on staff because of a real threat of redundancy while attempting to maintain quality assurance'.

To help staff cope with stress this hospital has support workers trained in listening skills, who refer when necessary to a team of trained counsellors. The role occupant perceived no real problems in the provider/purchaser/quality strategy based on a negotiated agreement of what the provider can realistically supply in order to meet the demands of the purchaser. There is a minimum of a yearly quality check on staff, but this normally happens more frequently. There are other built-in checks on the system, e.g. patient satisfaction questionnaires.

The manpower issues that are confronting the profession as a whole are a problem that needs to be addressed. The director stated 'We train too many nurses. This, coupled with frequent and major changes in the NHS, leads to problems in determining the requisite number of staff at any given time. This situation is rationalized by having a reserve of part-time nurses we call the "as and when" group, i.e. paid as and when they work. There is a nurse bank to cover the district'.

The Trust was considering the adoption of the 'clover leaf pattern' of employing nurses, which includes one third on permanent contracts, one third on fixed term contracts, and one third consisting of bank nurses. The director realized that this would affect Project 2000 students in terms of the nature of the contract offered on registration, but they were told before they commenced studentship that jobs were not guaranteed.

Project 2000 students in years 1 and 2 are supernumerary; year 3 students are rostered. When speaking about the training of Project 2000 students, the director stated 'UKCC and ENB policy is tantamount to expediency by trying to lift the "status" of nursing through a more academic training, rather than prepare them for the reality of their role in registration. They are too academically prepared. Ward sisters constantly complain that nurses are not prepared for the role and responsibilities of staff nurse'.

One area of concern to the director was that 'The RHA sees itself as the purchaser of education. Nurse directors have little influence other than being asked for views, which may or may not be subsequently addressed. We have minimal influence on preregistration education of nurses'. This lack of involvement and influence is economically unsound, because of the amount of money that needs to be spent out of tight budgets, giving nurses skills and knowledge that should have been given in preregistration training. To meet the needs of the new initiatives, all staff undertook in-house ongoing development, on a multidisciplinary basis. Individual performance review of all staff including nursing auxiliaries was compulsory.

My overall view of how this Trust was implementing the new initiatives is that they recognized the problems, worked together positively to overcome them and had built in monitoring and support procedures to ensure optimum quality.

In written communication from nurse executive directors in different parts of the country and in different waves of NHS Trusts, they expressed that there was a need to audit their quality initiatives; they perceived no detrimental effect on the delivery of care, although the only yardstick was the lack of complaints from patients. Most had no operational role and found difficulty at first in coping with this aspect. Stress levels were higher initially, but have been given ample opportunity to 'self-develop'. The role is developing; staff encountered more stress, which they attributed to change but they are now coming to terms with their new roles. No evaluation has been done to date to see how NHS Trusts are progressing.

Have nurses working for Hospital Trusts found greater favour in their role and enhancement of their conditions of employment? Or has this change adversely affected them, making their role and conditions of employment less attractive and more impoverished?

Nurses will continue to be required to care for patients. However, given that the many shortcomings of their present role together with the well-catalogued problems, including role overload, lack of appropriate skills and education to meet the demands of their job, stunted career prospects coupled with nurses' inability to provide a professional service and job uncertainty, especially for newly registered nurses, together trigger and compound nurses' stress, what, if anything, can a change in the status of individual hospitals provide to remedy the present anomalies? The perceived manpower cut-backs, uncertainty of tenure of employment, constriction of salary and the inevitable outcome of increased workload of existing staff, serve to compound and exacerbate existing problems.

The creation of Hospital Trusts, however limited or extensive, is seen by many as a leap forward, a change to improve the lot of patients and staff. However, some believe it to be a retrograde step, the first stage to privatizing the service. Is it a preface, at least for many vulnerable groups, including the elderly, the disabled, the mentally ill and the socially and economically impoverished, to the return of the state of health care prior to the much welcomed NHS? Or will the realization referred to by Butler (1992) come to fruition? 'The financial pressures upon the Hospital Trusts to dispense commercially unattractive services, however greatly they may be needed locally, negate the policy of meeting the full range of people's needs through the local district general hospital' (para. 1, p. 92).

Butler's theme seems in part to be substantiated by some of the comments from nurse executive directors, especially those relating to manpower problems and financial restrictions. There are also differences in the views of those interviewed as to whether the provider or purchaser dominate the negotiations in deciding priorities. It is not surprising that these differences arise, considering the magnitude of the change in nursing and the NHS and the relatively new and demanding role of the nurse executive director.

The time is now ready for nurses through their leaders, i.e. nurse executive directors, to adopt a positive attitude to ensure equal status in the boardroom, ensuring that nurses have a real voice in policy making and ensuring that standards and quality of care are not compromised in the interests of profit. Leadership is a dominant factor in the role of the nurse for the future. Nursing has for many years carried a lot of 'dead wood' and it must be eliminated. Many nurses have been content with basic qualifications, rarely updating their skills and knowledge to meet constant change. Most tend to blame the employer because of a lack of resources and never think of blaming themselves through lack of initiative. For example, computers are commonplace in hospitals and all local education departments run courses at very flexible times, but not many nurses avail themselves of the opportunity and say they are waiting for their employer to develop courses.

This is one of the most exciting and challenging times in the history of nursing and it is encumbent on nurses to seize every opportunity to develop and shape nursing so that it is a professional force to be reckoned with. To do this they will need to unite all sections of the profession and not lay bare their divisions, as stated in a report (DoH, 1989): 'Nursing represents a wide spectrum of professional interests and these divisions within the profession remain. Members of all three professions recognize what they themselves refer to as "tribalism". It is a strong element within their culture and they will take more than legislative change to remove it. A consequence of this is that the sectional interests, for individual members, take precedent over the more general professional interests and issues' (para, 2.10, p. 11).

Though difficult to forecast at this time, especially in the absence of any real evaluation, the role of the professional nurse will continue to be a demanding one. Traditionally, nurses have always wanted to care for patients, and no doubt will continue to do so, irrespective of the status of a hospital, but the effectiveness of the service they give will inevitably depend on their proper development, freedom to act and adequate support facilities pertinent to their identified needs. In this new ethos nurses must avoid a situation where they know the price of everything but the value of nothing. Taking on new initiatives does not mean that traditional values and standards, if they are high, must be discarded.

Nurses form a substantial core of the NHS workforce and as a direct result must be effectively prepared to meet the demands and responsibilities of this new era and play a major part in the fulfilment of their respective roles in the future success of these initiatives. In this context it is necessary to explore the following educational initiatives to establish the extent they can prepare nurses professionally for the demands of their future role.

Project 2000

There are obviously high hopes within certain factions of the nursing fraternity which, ever since the inception of Project 2000, have extolled in the absence of any full evaluation its virtues, especially heralding it as a long-awaited remedy, if not panacea, for the many and longstanding educational shortcomings of the profession. However, and not surprisingly, given the often repeated catalogue of rejection of many sound educational initiatives throughout the decades there exists within the profession a determined core of nurses, nurse educationists and nurse managers who, for diverse and sometimes unfounded reasons, vehemently oppose this initiative. This core of professionals may have sincere beliefs in the perceived inadequacies and/or inappropriateness of Project 2000 as the best way to prepare nurses in this century and beyond. However, the reality of the situation is that Project 2000 is already ongoing and, unless these professionals want this educational initiative to suffer the fate of the other sound ideas over the decades, they have to unite and endeavour to make it a success. As with all major change, no doubt Project 2000 may have flaws, but instead of dismissing the whole concept, professionals must remedy the inadequacies and strive for an educational foundation in nursing that is the best for nurses and patients receiving their care.

The 'negative' reasons, no doubt sincerely held and often made clear to me in the course of discussion by many nurses at different levels of the profession, tend to fall into two categories: social (status-related) and emotional (fear-related). Reasons that are social especially emphasize the educational, academic orientation of Project 2000, having the direct offshoot of producing a more academic type of nurse, rather than the more traditionally trained nurse, with a distinct practical or clinical orientation.

Nurses undertaking this initiative, apart from their personal motivation and attitude, are substantially influenced by the educationists responsible for their development, especially the academics in institutes of higher education, who play a major role in the development of nurses undertaking training under the aegis of Project 2000. Some of these may lack the necessary experience and knowledge of ward practice, sometimes being divorced from clinical practice for many years. In a recent comment, Hunt (1933) states: 'Nursing colleges are imposing misguided medically-dominated philosophical fads on their students in a misguided attempt to tackle poor quality care' (para. 1, p. 12). Is Hunt being realistic or purely provocative in these statements? If Hunt's concerns are realized this could seriously undermine the whole philosophy on which Project 2000 is based.

Some students currently undertaking this initiative also voice their fears. 'Lack of identity with the hospital including not belonging to any particular one, the situation being wholly impersonal' . . . 'Belonging to an amorphous group often without clear direction' . . . 'Fears of not securing a contract after training especially when our training only prepares us for nursing' . . . 'Most other graduates have a wider horizon and their courses can equip them for a choice of jobs'. This latter comment is supported by an officer of the RCN (in September 1993) who stated 'An increasing number of nurses are not given contracts, not even temporary contracts. There is an increase in the number of bank nurses which seems to be related to this occurrence'. These concerns are amplified by most of the executive nurse directors spoken to and interviewed.

On discussion with three large groups of Project 2000 students, they complained of 'Large gaps in our training that make us inadequate on the wards, even in our final years'; 'Our courses are badly designed and the curriculum does not equip us to meet the requirements of the *Code of Professional Conduct* or patients' needs'; 'Tutors say there is no time to fit in certain essential aspects of patient care, but on several days each week we have a lecture at 9.00 AM and nothing at all until 4.00 PM; we could use this time more usefully'; and 'The tutors never have enough time to explain things properly, we do not get handouts or course work returned at the times stated; the staff seem to be confused about the curriculum and often contradict each other'.

Many of these students were disillusioned and felt that the courses were not honouring the commitment given at interview. Some felt Project 2000 was 'a political expediency' and many felt that meeting patients' needs was 'unrealistic ideology'. The most worrying aspect of these discussions was the fact that most of the students thought the *Code of Professional Conduct* was 'just guidelines nurses should try to meet, but there are no repercussions if you do not' and that 'patients' rights are at the discretion of the nurse. It is quicker if you do not involve the patient'.

With the acceptance that this initiative is still in its early stages, these problems must not be allowed to continue unresolved, as they will be detrimental to yet another excellent educational initiative.

Project 2000 report (UKCC, 1986) represented the UKCC's views about the best way forward for the development of the education and training of nurses, midwives and health visitors. It was also a statement of the perceptions of the role of these practitioners and on their responsibilities in the delivery of care. The report acknowledged many shortcomings which in essence negate and/or undermine the traditional system. '. . . waste of resources in that students drop out of courses in large numbers; trained staff are not retrained; qualified nurses are not doing the work of nursing, instead they are outnumbered by students; and, there is a waste in the programmes that build on this flawed foundation' (para. 1.31, p. 13). The report having acknowledged these shortcomings, it identified the best way forward to include 'From the outset of their preparation, practitioners for the future will need to be better informed about the planning process, the information systems which feed it and the current policy debates which shape their work. The registered practitioner should be competent to engage in autonomous practice. Students should be supernumary to NHS staffing establishments throughout the period of preparation' (paras 2.37/2.40/5.44, pp. 20/44).

Currently there are 23 774 students undertaking Project 2000 programmes and 28 434 students undertaking traditional training programmes (ENB, 1993a). To date three research studies have been undertaken on Project 2000 by the National Foundation for Educational Research. The first study, *Charting the Course: A study of the 6 ENB Pilot Schemes in Pre-registration Nurse Education* (Leonard and Jowett, 1990), when dealing with the process of implementation, identified the following areas. A major outcome of the process of implementation was a thorough restructuring of management in the school of nursing. Greater autonomy for tutors was accompanied by greater accountability and it proved a difficult and lengthy process to get the balance right over who should decide what. Insufficient time and resources were identified as important factors impeding progress in every district. The time factor continued to be experienced as a problem throughout the operation of the pilot schemes, to some extent because of staff shortages. The supportive extended tutorial role also suffered from understaffing in the schools of nursing, so that tutor contact with ward staff and students during clinical practice was severely limited. The attitudes of existing staff who had received conventional training were a brake on the speed of assimilation of the new philosophy and limited the extent to which nurses could put it into practice. Senior training staff felt the new scheme had often been perceived as a threat. Ward sisters/charge nurses felt there was a conflict of interest; their main responsibilty for service delivery was at odds with their educational role. The abruptness of the shift from the school of nursing into the working situation was seen to contribute to student disorientation and vulnerability during clinical practice.

The researchers highlighted some of the solutions and strategies already in practice for addressing these identified problems. For example, all districts adopted initiatives to address the problem of inadequate initial preparation of both service and teaching staff by intensified training in assessment and mentorship; increased commitment and involvement of staff at all levels through the agency of new interorganizational management structures, e.g. inclusion of teaching staff in the decision making process; and some tutorial staff are endeavouring to spend more time in clinical settings in connection with student placements.

The second report (Jowett et al., 1991) stated as its main aim 'To provide an opportunity to learn from the experience of "first round" Districts as they take on the awesome task of implementing Project 2000' (para. 3, p. 1). Some concerns identified reflect a lack of adequate consultation and discussion which seems to arise from the limited time available and the extra demands by the course on people who already have an inordinate workload. Deadlines were set and imposed by the system of funding for Demonstration District Status which resulted in an acknowledged pragmatic and expedient approach. Initial teething problems could on reflection have a wider impact, e.g. the problems of dealing with large intakes of students. This has militated against a student-centred approach which is inherent in the philosophy of Project 2000. Additionally, much of the framework was not in place at the time deadlines needed to be met; even the lack of accommodation for such large intakes of students presented a major problem together with the lack of library resources (see also RCN, 1990).

The formal teaching of such large groups makes it difficult for lecturers/ tutors to take account of individual students' experience and education, especially when arranging placements. There are differences in the working patterns of staff in higher education and nursing education and these need to be clarified and negotiated. These findings are deemed by the authors of the report to be 'symptomatic of a widely expressed unease about what is on offer. Such unease peppered many of the interviews with teaching staff – sometimes starkly reinforced by comments such as "the students are getting the worst of both worlds"' (para. 2, p. 21). The report continues that even though there are many inadequacies the challenge for course providers must be 'to establish structures for collaborative working and provide opportunities for the airing of these difficulties' (para. 4, p. 21). The third report (Jowett *et al.*, 1992) was an interim report of a longitudinal study on Project 2000, of which the final report has recently been published (Jowett *et al.*, 1994).

Some issues discussed in this report include a sense of optimism about the potential of Project 2000 reforms for enhancing nursing education and practice together with the desire to rise to the challenge of an initiative of such magnitude. It was perceived that the potential links between nursing education and higher education were optimistically welcomed. However, this was tempered by some uncertainty about how to optimize the benefits of this far-reaching change.

There is still a need to address the problems of accommodation and course organization on some sites, as a matter of urgency, as well as the need to specify the anticipated purpose and outcome of the shorter placements, sometimes occurring in rapid sequence, with the possibility of replacing these with more extended placements. The authors of the report reflect the views stated throughout inerviews: 'Purveying information about Project 2000 throughout the nursing service, let alone allied disciplines, and preparing practice-based staff for their changed role was a Herculean task' (para. 2, p. 180). This lack of understanding of the broad philosophy of Project 2000 is leading to a confused and frustrating situation. Practice-based staff expressed 'surprise' at students' relatively limited practical skills. Some students spoke of 'fraught and confused encounters with staff in the practice areas about what they were able to do' (para. 3, p. 180). This situation may establish new frustrations for student nurses. They voiced their dilemma in having to 'negotiate their position on the spectrum of options "working to the college of nursing's protocol" and "working to a personal learning protocol"' (para. 1, p. 181).

In conclusion the report states: "There are varying degrees of caution urged in managing the fulfilment of these outcomes so that the appropriate balance is struck between the much-heralded improvements and the retention of the central tenets of nursing' (para. 4, p. 182).

The provision of learning experiences in the community summarized in a recent report (ENB, 1993b) stated 'The study found no evidence of resources or facilities being made available specially for supervisors in their work with Project 2000 students' (para. 7, p. 3). Many supervisors interviewed (number not given) commented 'for the most part, rooms were considered not important, because teaching was seen to take place on an informal basis, often in cars to and from visits' (para. 7, p. 3). If Project 2000 is to live up to its heralded reputation and expectations in reforming nursing education, this type of experience, in the name of expediency rather than educational experience, will only serve to damage and undermine the initiative.

The findings of these reports reflect in substance the findings of my own study as well as the concerns voiced by nurse executive directors and students undertaking Project 2000 training, during interview. These concerns should not be seen as a reflection on those involved with the initiative, but as an attempt to ensure that the concerns are very real and need to be addressed fully in order that Project 2000 becomes the success so deserved by nurses, the profession and the patients they serve.

FRAMEWORK FOR CONTINUING PROFESSIONAL EDUCATION AND HIGHER AWARD

The *Framework for Continuing Professional Education and Higher Award* is a major English National Board (ENB) initiative in continuing nursing education. The Framework is open to all and provides a flexible system for continuing professional education and a strucure leading to the ENB Higher Award, which is based on a partnership between practitioners, educationalists and managers. The Framework is identified by ten key characteristics which represent the areas of skill, knowledge and expertise which all practitioners must have in order to provide the quality of care needed to meet the health care needs of the general public. The ultimate ENB Higher Award is both a professional and academic award.

How it works

The Framework Higher Award incorporates a credit accumulation and transfer scheme (CATS) which enables practitioners to enter and leave the modular programme at times that suit them and their workload/commitment without losing recognition for the learning gained to that stage. A number of colleges of nursing and midwifery offering this programme have been approved by the ENB. The philosophy basically embodies a planned and focused approach to postregistration education; flexibility of professional development; balance between practical and academically oriented approaches; and enhanced links between colleges and institutes of higher education.

Comments on this initiative at this early stage are positive, supportive and welcoming. For example, Henry Foster (1992a), when commenting on how chief executives and general managers could help the implementation of this initiative, proposed:

> They should acknowledge the importance of investing in people and their skills; develop better means of identifying staff development requirements; plan inputs to support development programmes within existing resources and from new resources; develop an organisation culture which is supportive of staff development opportunities; and facilitate the necessary dialogues between purchasers, providers, and educational establishments to develop the use of the Framework.
>
> *(Paras 1/3, p. 2)*

In addition, Barbara Dixon (1992a) emphasized that:

> The 10 Key Characteristics that underpin the Framework and Higher Award give nursing a universal strategy for that development which encompasses professional development linked to clear clinical outcomes; quality specifics which can be linked to the contracting process; an effective recruitment, selection and retention strategy; clear benchmarks for workforce profiling; and individual performance review, a key to staff development and effective successive planning.
>
> *(Para. 5, p. 2)*

In a recent issue of ENB News (1992c) it was acknowledged that the initial enthusiasm for this initiative showed no sign of decreasing. One of the main attractions for practitioners and their managers is that the Higher Award offers both academic and professional recognition.

This initiative, long overdue, will hopefully go some way to correcting some of the present anomalies in nursing education at postregistration level. This remedy will only be successful if all staff are fully informed of its details and benefits together with adequate resourcing, especially proper study and library facilities. Staff undertaking this initiative will require support, encouragement and recognition.

The inherent partnership between practitioners, educationists and managers must be properly negotiated and its consequences fully understood in order to enable the flexibility and realization of this initiative. This negotiation between manager and practitioner must be based on performance review and realistically reflect nurses' needs and career aspirations as well as organization/patient/speciality needs.

However, enthusiasm, though rightly expressed must be tempered with caution in relation to the links between nursing colleges and institutes of higher education, many of which are undergoing major cuts in their resources, e.g. teaching staff and library provision. It is not realistic to expect such an improvement in standards without an increase in resources, and budgets must reflect this. In the absence of adequate financial resourcing, is it reasonable to expect nurses to fund in part or in total the cost of their professional development? Obviously nurses under the UKCC *Code of Professional Conduct* (1992; Para. 3) are required 'to maintain and improve [their] professional knowledge and competence'.

On discussion with some registered nurses regarding their aspirations and career development they commented 'I trained in the traditional way and have applied for a course to give me parity of qualifications with colleagues trained under Project 2000, but have been told it will cost me £400, and I cannot afford it'. 'I want to improve on my qualifications by undertaking courses that will enable me to be better equipped to do my job more efficiently and effectively, but am only allowed to go on courses I am sent on. I was never given the opportunity to negotiate or elect these courses and most of them are not even relevant'. 'I have a mortgage and a preschool child and cannot afford the course fees to undertake further development. The hospital seems to want a two-tier system of registered nurses; it does not augur well for a good working relationship'.

Managers and educationists need to reflect prior to selection of those seeking to undertake the Higher Award, and think about why they are sending somebody off and failing to plan for their return. This aspect is discussed in *Fortune* magazine (O'Reilly, 1993): 'No single approach to education works for every executive. Education should be a continuing process not a painful, one-time experience'. Managers should 'keep being sent back for more and make a point of capturing a freshly educated manager's insights as he or she grapples with new ideas or struggles to master a new way of doing things'. The article underlines that 'good companies don't just teach managers, they learn from them'. (©1993 Time Inc. All rights reserved.)

Management Today (Hackett, 1993), in an editorial which discussed the merits of MBAs, commented 'There is now much doubt about the value of the MBA degree – not least among MBAs themselves. One wonders where all the tutors from this massive infusion of business expertise came from. There is, too, the fact that training alone does not make successful managers. They need the inherent qualifications of character, a degree of self-subjugation, and above all, the ability to communicate and lead'. The essence of both these articles and the messages they contain for nurse practitioners and nurse managers is that the continuing educational development needs to be carefully planned, with clear objectives as to why staff are requesting or being sent on a particular course. More importantly, careful thought must be given in advance, by all parties concerned, as to what is expected of the person on completion of the course and recognize the fact that no particular course can totally equip the person to do their job. Managers must carefully monitor and evaluate the efficacy of a particular course in realizing their objectives. The curriculum framework included in the proposals of this text (Fig. 2) and its philosophy reflects the broad strategy in the ENB Framework.

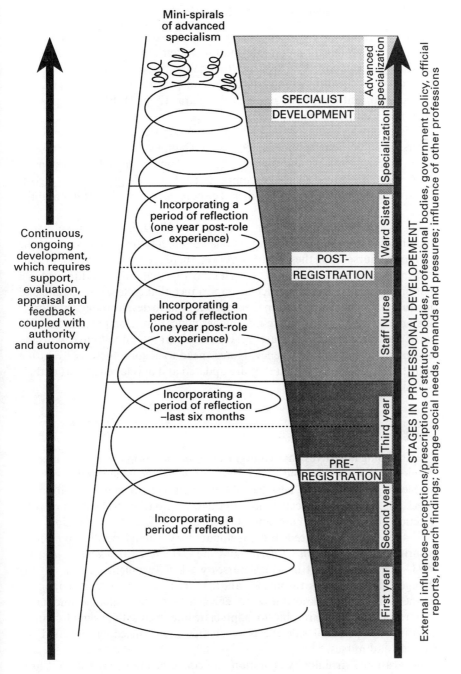

Fig. 2 The spiral curriculum: progressively linked stages in professional development.

ENB Campus: communication and information

Basic to any effective educational system is a sound, usable and readily available communication and information system. In this respect, the ENB (1992a) has established a system 'to enable those working in nursing, midwifery and health visiting education and practice to communicate and access important data bases more easily' (para. 12, p. 3). ENB Campus is a section of Campus 2000.

Using software, students and teachers can connect their own microcomputers through the telephone system to the Campus 2000 service. Users can select, retrieve, process and use information from Campus 2000's extensive data bases. Electronic mail and computer conferencing give access to cost-effective communication with other Telecom Gold users throughout the world.

There is a comparable system, namely JANET (Joint Access Network), already in existence. However, questions are already being asked about the cost to the nurse using these systems. As yet, there are no answers, but in view of the potential value of these systems, it is an area that must be addressed as a matter of urgency. It is of particular importance that colleges of nursing and institutes of higher education, in their negotiations to develop courses, address this area as more nurses move into higher education. Computer use and in particular access networks are very much part of an effective working environment that seeks efficiency. Nurses need to acquire these skills during basic training and ensure that they are updated and developed as part of their continuing education.

Change

The foregoing initiatives have embodied in their philosophy major change for the nurse, the profession, the NHS organization and the patient. All have faced problems arising out of new technology, restricted resources, manpower issues, e.g. increased specialization and new approaches to work and work practices, many of which are embodied in, and prefaced by, legislation.

Change is also prefaced and precipitated by altered public opinion as enshrined in *The Patient's Charter* and the *NHS and Community Care Act 1993*. The environment in which nurses work is turbulent because of this change. In view of this turbulence and its effects, it is vital that managers, teachers and nurses know how to effect and manage change and most important that they are able to appreciate the events that signal change, ensuring the personal side-effects of change are reduced or obviated for patients and nurses.

Innovations, virtually by definition, are concerned not only with unlearning, but most importantly with increased learning and relearning, on an individual and/or group basis. This increased learning and relearning is central to understanding one's new role and being fulfilled by it through job confidence, security, educational enlightenment and the enhancement of the quality of care.

Innovation and change is about how to introduce new ideas, personally, organizationally, managerially, educationally and clinically, and to change existing structures and philosophies. Some nurses may feel inadequate to initiate or influence change in a positive way, because of their position in the organization and/or because of their lack of knowledge, skills or expertise; or because of their lack of interest.

Regrettably, sometimes the reasons underlying change may not be made known to staff, or if they are known they may not seem to be relevant to the improved efficiency of their working. Also, little if any preparation of staff may have taken place, thus accentuating this bewilderment as well as possibly increasing their stress due to apprehension or anxiety about the nature of the intended change together with its consequences for them, i.e. apprehension about their changing role, new demands (physically and emotionally), loss of status and possible redundancy. Central to introducing change is an attempt to influence the behaviour of people, preferably in a desired and planned way. Therefore, it is wise for management to recognize and consider important aspects, such as communication, ensuring staff are fully informed of the nature and effects of the change contemplated and participation (people follow their own decisions best). The intended change must seem relevant and essential to the improved functioning of the profession/organization. Management has the responsibility of encouraging, motivating and supporting staff during the preparatory period and during the phase of actual change. The importance of this is underlined by Fulmer (1988), who states 'When attitudes are being changed, it is necessary to eliminate, or unfreeze, the present attitudes so that a vacuum can be created for new ones'. He also urges managers to identify staff within the organization who are opinion leaders, who share the values of the intended change and who are able to identify with and influence others. In essence they become change agents. The profession, the organization and managers must acquire much-needed marketing skills and present new initiatives in a way that will attract people who will want to make them work; ensure that all the facts are given to ensure that people do not feel let down when the changes take place; give people the opportunity to assess what is on offer and the choice of whether or not they want to stay and be part of it; ensure forums of participants for feedback.

The resistance to change may occur for many reasons, of which innovators must be aware and which they must if possible obviate or diminish. The many impediments to change include inconvenience; the working environment may be more difficult; new ideas and attitudes have to be acquired and new information effected, possibly through new learning or unlearning; new approaches are full of uncertainty and individuals feel threatened; social and working relationships may be affected through staff adopting different approaches; and resentment, if the change comes solely from management without consultation of staff. Resentment may well accentuate resistance to the intended change.

Innovation and change offer both a challenge to one's creativity, inventiveness and managerial prowess, and a threat to one's personal security. Managers must be aware that change can show a marked increase in staff stress and must have in place counselling and support systems before change is introduced in order to minimize its damaging effect. In this way both innovation and change can be less emotionally taxing and traumatic for those responsible for providing the innovation and masterminding the change, as well as for the recipients of change. The whole process of managing major change requires the skills of planning, motivating and educating staff as well as the skill of managing change. In addition, it requires knowledge, tact, interest, commitment, support and the perseverance of managers and staff.

Much has been published relating to the change process, how to introduce it and its effects on staff, including works by Bennis (1966), Drucker (1980), Cooper (1981), Mauksch and Miller (1981), Argaris (1985), Mangham (1988), Loveridge and Pitt (1990) and Twiss (1992). These publications may be of value to the reader when looking at the principles of change. However, nothing to date has been written to examine the huge task of implementing the vast range of change currently happening in the nursing profession and health services as a whole.

PART TWO

PROPOSALS AND CURRICULUM IMPLICATIONS

In light of the foregoing analysis of the role of the professional nurse, the following proposals are made by way of offering possible corrective measures which in time, if earnestly addressed, might alleviate or obviate some of the identified shortcomings which, to a greater or lesser extent, affect the operation of the professional nurse's role. The proposals are in the main related to the findings of the original study (Bowman, 1990), together with current research into the major elements of new initiatives in nursing and the health service which affect this role. Some are not new and have been identified in the literature on role-related research over many decades. However, often for reasons unclear and despite the integrity of the sources, they continue to be stubbornly unaddressed.

NURSES' ROLE AND RELATED ELEMENTS

Many nurses experienced difficulty during interviews in understanding concepts which are basic to their role:

Management
They viewed management in general terms and had difficulty grasping its core elements, e.g. leadership, planning, co-ordinating, motivating, evaluating, monitoring, assessing and appraising.

Administration
The word 'administration' was seen as being synonymous with management and was largely viewed as form-filling and paperwork generally.

Nursing
Nursing was interpreted virtually entirely in terms of direct patient care rather than the global care of the patient, meeting all their needs.

Evaluation
This was seen largely in subjective, visual terms despite having patient care plans, rather than in objective, criteria-based terms.

Authority
There was confusion in nurses' responses as to the nature of their authority. Nurses assumed that authority was inherent in their professional role, though there was little evidence of them possessing real authority in the management of their role, including key functions of resource acquisition and in some instances the management of patient care.

Autonomy
They viewed autonomy as being synonymous with authority.

Accountability
This was rarely seen in the context of the UKCC *Code of Professional Conduct*. They seemed to think that personal accountability was transferable. They had difficulty separating responsibility from accountability.

Nurses generally perceived their role differently from the perceptions of their bosses. They acknowledged a role which is essentially a 'caring/nursing' one. In contrast, nurse managers perceived the nurses' role as being 'substantially managerial/administrative' in nature, especially the role of the ward sister, with a prescribed teaching element. They perceived the role of ward sister and staff nurse as being virtually interchangeable in respect of duties, tasks, responsibilities and accountability. The problem that emerges is that nurses are essentially prepared for their nursing role and only a limited extent, if at all, for the managerial/administrative demands of their role. This inadequacy should have been addressed by Project 2000. However, during discussions with nurse executive directors, staff nurses and ward sisters the situation was found to remain relatively unaddressed. Newly qualified nurses said 'We have not been prepared for such a sudden takeover of these major responsibilities', and 'You do not expect to be left in charge so soon. There was nothing in my training to prepare me for this; it terrifies me'.

The role of the nurse has changed, but it would appear that the new initiatives designed to meet the needs of this new role are not keeping up with the range of change that is needed. Nurses have little control over the events for which they are held accountable. This, coupled with the fact that nurses perceive management and administration to some extent as alien to their role, compounds the problem and potentially affects their ability in the execution of that role.

The first thing nurses need to do is endorse the new policies and initiatives and not be shortsighted, be more transparent and more co-operative, because concentrating on disillusionment helps no-one. They need to move away from the micro detail and look at the macro effect.

The grey and often disputed areas of the professional nurses' role must be clearly defined so that nurses know whether they are able to cope with their role. Often job descriptions are out of date and unrealistic. When hospitals altered their status to NHS Trusts many of the incumbent staff retained their role, but it was clear from discussions with some nurses and nurse executive directors that these staff took on a more demanding role. However, in many instances, it was only after the event that the training for this change was instigated. This framework, which would have enabled nurses to take on the responsibilities of the new initiatives with certainty and security, should have been in place in preparation for this initiative. Nursing, in the past, despite the attempts of Salmon (1966) and Griffiths (1983) to impose a managerial structure, substantially failed in preparing nurses for the demands of their role.

The time is long overdue for a radical reappraisal of the job of the nurse. During the study of the nurses' role there were some disparities identified between the behaviours prescribed and embodied in nurses' job descriptions, the behaviours assumed by nurses and stated during interview to be present in their job, and behaviours observed during periods of observation. In this context, there is a need to examine their manifest role, their prescribed, agreed job; their role, activities assumed to be present in their role by nurses themselves and nurse managers, including their duties, their responsibilities, accountability and related authority and autonomy; and their extant role, the actual behaviours shown through systematic analysis.

To facilitate this, a job analysis needs to be undertaken in order to determine the purpose, scope, responsibilities and tasks of the nurses' role, together with a serious acknowledgement of job design to establish specification of job requirements in order to satisfy and address current and future technological and organizational demands as well as the social and personal needs of the nurse.

In effect, the reality of the nurses' job needs to be established now and as envisaged in the future and decisions need to be made on the relevant skills and knowledge and the best educational framework within which these can be developed. If, as at present, the nurses' role has major elements of managerial, administrative, teaching, communication, finance and budgetary control, then in the interest of efficiency of the service together with the confidence, security and job satisfaction of the role occupant, these must be realistically addressed, not just in theoretical debate but more importantly in practical application. Where are nurses to obtain these skills? Is the NHS the best place to gain these skills, if one takes into account that the NHS has moved from being an organization whose nursing staff knew the price of nothing, to becoming an organization whose nursing staff need to know the price of everything? This concept has been much maligned, with many people thinking, wrongly, that it is all about money instead of the fact that it is about obtaining the best service for patients in an efficient and effective way. Postregistration nurses could be offered training on an in-house basis, which would develop individuals to take on their new role with its incumbent responsibilities and accountability. There may be a need to engage appropriate expertise as and when required. Job rehearsal could be introduced as an option of giving registered nurses, at all levels, the opportunity to obtain experience of doing the next-level job, for a mutually agreed time by management and the nurse, without any contractual agreements binding on the employer or employee.

During this period of experience, nurses would gain valuable skills, including interactive skills, making them effective with peers or other professionals and sensitive to the reasons for the behaviours of their peers and others. This experience could be further advanced by use of group dynamics or 'T-groups'. However, these groups need to be conducted by a specialist in this field and very carefully monitored.

The added advantage of job rehearsal enables the individual to experience, albeit to a lesser degree, the demands of the job, and more importantly can tell the individual whether or not they can meet the demands of their own aspirations. It will also help identify for the nurse and management the inadequacies in skills and knowledge that need to be addressed before that particular level of job can be a reality for the person concerned. All staff should be prepared in advance of taking up post to ensure confidence and competence, in the interest of quality patient care.

Project 2000 studentship could be a four-year sandwich course with a middle year on placement in industry in order for the necessary industrial/business ethic to be acquired. It would also benefit the student in the long term by broadening their experience and offering wider job opportunities, in light of current uncertainty and contractual limitations of full employment of all nurses.

If this proposition is considered in respect of the potential and positive effects to the nurse and the profession, students' aspirations could change, e.g. instead of their intention to 'nurse and care for people' they could turn that intention to a positive 'care and nurse patients in an efficient and effective way'. (These ideas will be explored further in the proposal on professional development.)

High upon the priorities of managers should be the objective of enabling and ensuring nurses' job satisfaction. To enable this, there must be an enrichment of the nurses' job through the provision of greater freedom to act and make decisions; greater responsibility must be matched with the requisite authority to promote improved performance and motivate staff and in this way reduce some of the tensions identified by nurses and relating to these elements of their job.

Present guidelines within which professional nurses operate, identified in the document *Scope of Professional Practice* (UKCC, 1992) and *Boundaries of Nursing* (RCN, 1988) are useful, but are they heeded by nurses and nurse managers? In this context, nurses must have clear-cut boundaries within which to practise and make day-to-day decisions on matters relating to the care of their patients and the management of their wards. This must inevitably mean nurses having greater involvement in policy-making which affects their wards, especially in terms of its resourcing.

Nurses must acknowledge any shortcomings in their training and insist on these being addressed, if they feel they cannot cope with the demands of their new role. Good, effective communication, support systems and interpersonal relationships between nurses and their managers are imperative to the effective, efficient operation of the nurses' role. To enable effective communication and representation of the views of staff, a consultative committee is required at ward/speciality level, with all staff choosing a representative at their grade. This ward committee would then select a member to represent them at a higher level of negotiation, e.g. the nurse executive director. The staff at ward level will have the satisfaction of knowing their views are being heard. For communication to be successful it has to be a two-way process. The ward staff will receive replies from the senior nurse management through their own representatives. This system has the added benefit of being a catalyst for new ideas and a means of ensuring the effective dissemination of information.

Where there is strong and comprehensive accountability inherent in the nurses' role these must be met with the commensurate authority, which must include the rights of appointment of subordinate staff; rights to make significant alterations in individual responsibility, according to how the nurse performs in practice; rights to set general directions as well as specific tasks; and, the right to deselect staff who are found to be unsuitable. In this context, a decision must be made on the type of authority relationship embodied in the role of the ward sister. It must be made clear as to whether it is intended to be a main-line managerial relationship which, in addition to the prescribed duties of the role occupant in Rowbottom's (1987) view must include the authority to initiate 'promotion, transfer and dismissal' (para. 3, p. 11), or 'a supervisory relationship which does not include authority for the latter' (para. 2, p. 12).

The role of the ward sister, which is assumed to be mainly managerial, needs to be clarified, to decide whether the role is main-line managerial or supervisory, otherwise it becomes impossible for the role occupant to maintain the integrity of their professional role, and for appropriate preparation to take place. It is good that nursing has a vision of the role of the nurse, but visionaries who only see the horizon, without dealing with the obstacles and inadequacies along the way, will never reach the horizon.

The principal publications dealing with the role of the nurse include those of Hardy and Conway (1978), Pembrey (1980), DoH, Nursing Division (1989), RCN (1988), UKCC (1992) and the Audit Commission (1991, 1992).

STANDARD AND QUALITY OF CARE

The evidence of the study shows the difficulty many nurses experience in ensuring the standard and quality of care for which they are accountable. This point was emphasized during the study in a statement by an officer of one of the nursing statutory bodies when certain problems were acknowledged in the standard and delivery of care: 'High standards of care can only be provided if the workforce is stable, properly qualified and well motivated'.

Reasons often given by nurses for their inability to offer a quality service to their patients included those relating to the inadequacy of manpower resources and facilities, the wrong mix of skills, the frequent use of agency nurses to fill gaps and a heavy reliance on nursing auxiliaries. This they linked to their inability to regulate the workload on colleagues and subordinates. To improve the quality and standards of care, a thorough analysis of the role of each member of the ward team needs to be carried out by a member of management, to identify what they do, how they do it, why they do it in that way and how long it takes.

Nurses must be prepared in their final year of training, which is advanced on appointment as staff nurse, in time management and staff management including staff utilization and support. This enables a team approach to patient care to be put on a more effective basis that includes the proper use of resources and facilities.

Care systems must be agreed and used consistently and not only when it is convenient, so that all members of the ward team are fully acquainted with the clinical condition, treatment and care of all patients. This is desirable, even though patients have a 'named nurse' responsible for their care, who may, for many reasons, be absent from the ward.

Even though most hospitals appear to have a nurses' bank, a pool of nurses attached to a speciality could be more advantageous. The ward sister could have a resource of suitably trained, experienced nurses established on a rotation basis, who would be available as back-up as and when the need arose. A smaller pool, as opposed to the larger bank, has the advantage of being readily accessible, can relate to the needs of the speciality and improve continuity.

The patient must always be the focus of ward activity, they and their relatives being involved as far as practicable in their care programme. Nurses must ensure that the instruments available to them for patient assessment, workload assessment, monitoring and evaluating care and the information provided are made readily available to the ward team. The evaluation of patient care must be objectively done using stated and agreed criteria, in order that standards and quality can be readily established, updated and revised as necessary. This has the added advantage of establishing parity in the quality and standard of care.

Nurses must be trained in the skills of assessing and evaluating, listening, communicating and identifying patients' needs; once acquired, the skills must be used. The professional development of nurses must be viewed not only in terms of career progression but also in the context of nurses keeping up-to-date with educational, technological and clinical developments which if deemed appropriate are acted upon, thus ensuring that the care given to the patient is always the best available.

The Audit Commission report (1992) identified three main problems which affect the quality of nursing care and need to be addressed: 'a lack of systematic approaches to quality assessment and quality improvement; a need to bring responsibility for care and control of ward resources much closer together; and a need for greater clarity in management roles and relationships, particularly those of ward sisters and their immediate superiors' (para. 57, pp. 27/28). This view was often repeated by nurses during interviews.

In addition to what has already been stated under standards and quality of patient care, there is much more which underpins this, and needs to be addressed. This includes courtesy to patients, e.g. welcoming new patients, being friendly and not officious, talking and listening to what they say and getting to know them as individuals and respecting their privacy, confidentiality and dignity. This would substantially lessen the formality of ward practice and procedure and encourage patients' confidence and security. The care plan can be an excellent medium for establishing and ensuring this, really getting the patient and their relatives involved and reducing the mystique and fear which patients often associate with being in hospital. This can only truly work in the interest of the patient and the nurse, if nurses accept the principle of patients' rights and patients' participation and feel free to act and manage resources enabling greater flexibility of their discretion and better use of their time.

The literature on standards and quality of care, associated problems and suggested remedies includes that of Briggs (1972), Merrison (1979), Moores and Thompson (1986) and the National Audit Office (1985).

PATIENTS' ROLE AND PATIENTS' NEEDS

Today's National Health Service is patient-led with emphasis placed on patient participation and consultation. The *Patient's Charter* (DoH, 1991) embodies the rights of patients, what they should expect from health services and what to do if it is not forthcoming. The charter also seeks to raise the standard and quality of care given to patients. It intends that the patient is always put first and the services provided meet local and national standards in ways responsive to people's views and needs. Health authorities must publish and make available their own local charter standards.

During the study, nurses stated 'There is little, if any, involvement of patients or their relatives in their care programme', as this enabled them to get things done much quicker. One nurse manager stated 'The patient does not have a role'. During periods of observation, there was much evidence to support the lack of real involvement of the patient. Even though care plans were drawn up, this was only done in a very subjective way and was rarely drawn upon after initial admission. Care planning appeared to be an expediency, it helped with case history information, there was little dialogue but much note-taking by preoccupied nurses. Very little in-depth discussion or evaluation of patient care took place, the sessions were brief and sometimes hurried and frequently interrupted, they gave little time for discussion and understanding of the patient or their views and needs and it was mainly task-related, routine and ritualistic.

Nurses need a change of attitude; they must understand the patient-led philosophy. The patient must be allowed to identify their needs and nurses must be prepared to meet those needs. The patients' role and patients' needs are intrinsically linked. There must be a reawakening and realization in nurses and nurse managers of the relevance and centrality of patients and their relatives to any successful care programme ensuring patient involvement, not just as an acquiescence to some imposed system or process of care thought to be useful, but intrinsically realizing the value of a particular approach in enabling patients and their relatives to share in the decision-making about their care. In this way some of the mystique that surrounds nursing/clinical practice can be removed. This approach would contribute considerably to reduce the patient's fear and anxiety, accelerate their recovery and make their stay in hospital more acceptable.

Emphasis must be placed on patients' individuality with individual needs, which must always be given priority over questionable ward routines and practice, no matter how important these may be deemed to the 'smooth' running of the ward. To enable this the role of nurse management involves leadership and motivation of nurses, provision of the necessary facilities and ensuring the right atmosphere and clinical environment. Central to this is a close nurse/patient relationship.

The patient must be given a clear explanation of any treatment proposed, any risks involved and any alternatives available, before they agree to any treatment. Special care and expertise will be required to ensure that patients with sensory handicap and others with communication or learning difficulties are able to access and understand the information given. Patients must be made aware of their right to access their health records and be able to choose whether or not they wish to take part in medical research or medical student training. The patient must be told that they have the right to choose the consultant by whom they wish to be treated and if necessary they can be referred for a second opinion.

Nurses must respect the privacy, dignity and religious and cultural beliefs of the patient. They must ensure that practical arrangements are made for dietary requirements. Private rooms must be provided for confidential discussions with relatives. Nurses must ensure that they understand and are able to identify the needs of people with a disability. Nurses must ensure that they are able to communicate with people with sensory handicap and ensure that the ward has facilities that will enable friends and relatives to obtain information regarding the patient's progress, e.g. a minicom telephone on each ward to enable the profoundly deaf to make enquiries.

Finally, nurses need to ensure that continuing health and social needs of the patient are met before discharge from hospital. They need to make themselves fully aware of the support agencies that will benefit the patient on discharge. Nurses must consult with the patient and their carers at every stage of health care and ensure that there is joint decison-making.

In the study, many impediments were perceived by nurses, which readily prevented them fully meeting patients' needs. These can be summarized as manpower-related, skill-related, time-related, role-related and educationally related. In essence, these are lack of ward staffing, continued use of inexperienced and/or unqualified staff, the inappropriate placement of nurses, mainly agency nurses, lack of proper professional development and updating and inordinate workload. Action needs to be taken to address these inadequacies.

Patients are empowered by the *Patient's Charter* to demand that their needs are met, but how can this realistically be done in light of the inadequacies? Each of the identified categories of impediment needs to be addressed. For example, ward staffing levels need to be examined to determine whether there are staff shortages, or whether staff are being wrongly deployed in terms of their skills and expertise, and to establish whether ward support facilities, e.g. ward clerks, are needed to relieve professionally trained nurses of clerical tasks.

Managers must identify where skill shortages are and address them as a matter of urgency, e.g. by creation of care plans, nurses must have the basic skills of communication, listening, assessing and evaluating as well as the speciality skills of British Sign Language. They will also require a knowledge of rehabilitative medicine, support services and how to co-operate with other agencies. The skill mix and the skill inadequacies in the individual need to be dealt with as separate issues. The former can be addressed by establishing the clinical demands and the nature of the workload of the particular ward or speciality; the latter requires an effective and ongoing educational programme which makes it compulsory for staff to address identified skill deficiencies. Professional development in this respect must be deliberate and continuing and address the diversity of competencies related not only to the present, but also to the future work tasks of nurses. This must be arranged in concert with the nurse, the manager and the individual's colleagues. Both purchasers and providers have an interest in the avoidance of nurse incompetence.

Time management needs to be evaluated on a regular basis. Nurses need to look at how they organize and manage their workload, tasks and the team and be advised on improved ways of time management, allocating, deciding, effecting, monitoring, appraising and evaluating the work to be done and ensuring that appropriate use is made of the skills and competence available. Staff performance needs to be regularly monitored with a view to effecting improvements and change when indicated.

Role overload requires analysis of the job of the nurse including its duties and tasks to establish the nature, extent and reality of the workload. This will identify whether the perceived overload is incurred because of the inability of the role occupant to manage the required workload effectively through a lack of training and expertise, or whether there is an actual overload. If the problem is properly identified then action can be taken. Inadequacies that are identified as a lack of training and/or development must be addressed in an ongoing educational programme.

For the *Patient's Charter* to have any meaning, these anomalies need to be remedied as identified in the Audit Commission report (1992), which links the continuity of patient care and patient-centred care with the full utilization of ward resources, including the proper use of support staff time 'to release nursing time for patients' (para. 22, p. 15). Patient-related research and literature on role and needs has been identified in Chapters 3 and 7.

RESOURCES AND FACILITIES

In the study many nurses stated there was an under-staffing in particular, and an under-resourcing and lack of facilities generally, of their wards. In the main this view was confirmed during periods of observed behaviour and to an extent was supported by nurse managers.

There is no national policy despite much research on the effective staffing of wards and this needs to be remedied. Nurses must have more say in the resourcing of wards; there must be a closer link between how wards are managed and resourced. This is beginning to happen within NHS Trust hospitals, where ward sisters have been given responsibility for the ward budget. In this context the ward sister has the responsibility for interviewing and selecting registered nurses, though to date they have little if any real control on the allocation of nursing students to their wards. Ward sisters need the authority to remove nurses they feel are not efficient or effective. Currently, the final censure of dismissal lies with the senior nurse manager and/or nurse executive director; the ward sister can only advise and recommend.

There must be relevant, appropriate training for support staff. Where systems whether manual or computerized are employed to assess manpower needs and skill mix, these must be used efficiently and effectively and be constantly updated and regularly monitored. Information must be disseminated to all staff concerned and not just managers.

There needs to be continuity of the ward team and much more careful thought and deliberation given to the constitution and continued stability of the ward team, with particular emphasis on appropriate skill mix. This necessitates having an effective policy in relation to dealing with *ad hoc* deficiencies that may occur in relation to the staff of a particular ward. The borrowing of nurses from other wards and the casualness of deploying bank and/or agency nurses must be eradicated. Evidence in the study showed much frustration and anger by nurses over this issue, which they felt was based on expediency, a lack of planning and a lack of appreciation of the potential effects on staff thus involved. Staff nurses who were often moved to another ward, even though they were not familiar with that ward or its routines, felt it was done because the ward needed a nominal figurehead of a registered nurse in charge, irrespective of whether or not he/she could be effective.

The ward sister must identify the skills and knowledge inadequacies in her staff and have a voice in ensuring they receive the necessary training to remedy this situation.

Planners must ensure adequate facilities to meet patients' needs. Currently, planners seem only to address what is required by regulation and legislation and do not address the most effective and efficient aspects of the final results. They look at legislation relating to the building without regard to the inherent problems it presents in not meeting other criteria. For example, the *Patient's Charter* requires nurses to respect the privacy, dignity and confidentiality of patients, yet planners still design bedspace divided by flimsy curtains, in multi-million pound projects. Planners still think of access as a ramp, not taking into account colour contrasting of bathroom fixtures, exits, entrances, etc., which would enable real access. The list is endless, and nurses should have a stronger voice in the planning and design of hospitals.

Further research in a DHSS report (1983) identifies several issues relating to nurse manpower on which more study might be profitable and on which little has been done, including 'Evaluation of the cost of employing different manpower, e.g. full/part timers and agency staff as well as identifying, monitoring and recording absence, sickness, and wastage rates in order to devise strategies for control and as a management tool for planning the allocation of staff' (paras 5.30/5.33, pp. 7/8).

It is important that there is a more equitable distribution of resources, manpower and facilities, throughout all clinical specialities. Longstay wards appear to be particularly impoverished in relation to registered nurses and facilities, and this bears no relation to the needs of the patients, many of whom may have benefited from professional expertise.

The intention of management must be to ensure a system which enables optimum use of the abilities, skills, knowledge, initiative and creativity of nurses at each level of the organization, encouraging their participation and/or reducing their underdeployment and in this way improving individual job satisfaction, as well as furthering the cost-effectiveness of the organization.

Other research and literature includes that by the National Audit Office (1985), the DoH, Nursing Division (1989), the Audit Commission (1991) and Seccombe and Buchan (1993).

These proposals are intended to heighten the focus of some of the problems perceived to be inherent in the role of the professional nurse and evidenced in the text. Many of these problems are dated. However, they continue despite the introduction of corrective initiatives, including those that are educational in nature, and are now well established.

The proposals are interrelated organizationally, educationally and operationally as regards the nature of the organization and the environment, hospital or ward in which work is undertaken, including job elements, job satisfaction and job enrichment. The proper development of the nurse in the skills required in the performance of their job and nurses' ability to operate with confidence and security under the umbrella of appropriate authority and autonomy are central to the integrity of the nurses' role and the resulting quality of the service to their patients. The proposals, if properly targeted, would go some way to correcting deficiencies and/or anomalies in the person and in the organization, through improved communication, consultation and participation with staff at all levels of management and by their improved education. Basic to the successful implementation of these proposals is the agreement and formulation of an appropriate educational policy and philosophy that embraces the entire career development of the nurse.

EDUCATIONAL PHILOSOPHY: FRAMEWORK FOR IMPLEMENTATION

Continuing education if it is to be effective must enable the nurse to acquire, develop and continually update the basic competencies as defined in the

Nurses, Midwives and Health Visitors Rules Approval Order 1983 (paras 18/24/35/39). In addition, continuing education must take account of the special needs of nurses that relate to their career enhancement, special and/or new and more demanding responsibilities and working relationships.

Education and training, to be of value, must be continually developed, appraised, evaluated and updated. The success of continuing education and staff development relies substantially on the nature and quality of the educational opportunities which are provided at the place of work as well as other factors, especially those relating to the selection and ongoing appraisal of staff.

Basic nursing education can only be a foundation, but that foundation needs to be properly balanced and form a firm basis on which to build a programme of continuing education. It needs to be followed up by systematic and more advanced preparation of nurses for specialized roles through a process of carefully planned, postregistration educational programmes which must involve the nurses, nurse managers and nurse educationalists, in order to satisfy the needs of the individual, the organization, the profession and the patient. Staff development in this context is the intentional, continuing enhancement of many and different competencies. It is not purely self-development.

No single learning process, if the educational process is to be effective, seems adequate on its own. In this respect a number of factors affect the choice of learning methods, which include the nature of learning, the learner's learning style, the teacher's learning style, the resources available, the motivation of staff to learn, the environment in which learning takes place and the way educational programmes are marketed.

The level of learning, e.g. memory, understanding, application and transfer, will vary with the learning methods whether these be off-the-job, including lectures, talks, programmed learning, discussion, role play, experimental learning, group exercises and sensitivity training, or on-the-job, which includes assignments, projects, job rotation, job rehearsal, supervised practice and discovery learning.

In order to learn, nurses must want to learn. Essentially, learning is enhanced when people perceive a reason for learning; therefore, it is of vital importance that nurses are made aware of the significance and relevance of continuing education. Continuing education must embrace all staff, and if necessary with an element of compulsion, otherwise if offered in an informal way only the 'converted' will accept the offer, whilst the problem of poor performers is never addressed.

To enable staff development to be an effective reality the following points must be addressed:

• The acquisition of competencies must be treated on an equitable basis, not attaching particular prestige to one over another.

- The creativity, skills, abilities and talents of nurses must be identified, encouraged and developed through proper assessment, counselling and support systems.
- Staff must not in any way feel alienated from the mainstream of education, or be the victims of cynicism.
- Nurse managers must provide proper leadership and in this respect must ensure that staff deficiencies are recognized, highlighted and addressed.
- Positive attitudes must be encouraged to reduce fear and develop staff confidence.
- The culture of the ward, hospital and district must be responsive, imaginative and encouraging, provide clear values, create trust and confidence and make staff feel valued.

If these measures are adopted, they would go some way to enabling staff to meet their obligations as stated in the *Code of Professional Conduct* (UKCC, 1992): 'Maintain and improve your professional knowledge and competence' and 'acknowledge any limitations in your knowledge and competence and decline any duties and responsibilities unless able to perform them in a safe and skilled manner' (paras 3/4).

Project 2000 was intended to address many of these anomalies in its stated principles:

> Ensure a lifelong progression of professional learning; provide a simpler and less costly overall result; enhance a sense of unity and integration among those who practise in nursing, midwifery and health visiting; and, achieve all this without sacrificing the real strengths of the current pattern of specialisation. The aim is to produce a different practitioner, via a very different pattern of preparation and under conditions for teaching and learning which will be a long way from those which at present obtain.
>
> *(Paras 6.2/6.8, p. 45)*

The intention is fine in principle, but until the full circle evolves and all nurses are trained under the aegis of Project 2000, there remains the deficiency that exists amongst postregistration staff, and this requires urgent remedy. Added to this is the reality that many Project 2000 students are perceived by many ward sisters and some executive nurse directors to be 'too theoretically trained and not well prepared for the role of staff nurse especially in the practicalities of running a ward'.

This does not indicate that we should abandon Project 2000; many initial problems will be sorted out; but there must be serious acknowledgement of any deficiencies and notice taken of any ongoing evaluation and its recommendations, otherwise the integrity of the entire concept is at risk.

Nurses' low status and submissiveness, which emanate from nursing tradition and social iniquity, must be changed by sound, effective educational practice. During interviews and discussions with nurses they were found to perceive their training and/or ongoing development to lack:

- preparation in administrative and managerial skills and knowledge;
- the skills of counselling, teaching, communication and interpersonal relating, especially with staff, patients and relatives;
- resource management and manpower management, including planning, organizing, leading, motivating and supervising;
- proper discussion, participation and negotiation relating to their development.

There were differences of opinion amongst the nurses as to when they should undergo the development of these skills, i.e. last year of studentship (64%), on completion of basic training but prior to registration (32%) or a few (4%) after one year in post. However, none advocated the concept of professional development taking place from the beginning of studentship and continuing throughout their professional career.

In any reorganization or rationalization of nursing education, the position of students is paramount. They will become the future professionals – nurses, teachers and managers. Their development must be taken seriously, and is beginning to be with Project 2000, and so serve as a blueprint for the future of the profession. This means without equivocation ensuring controlled professional development, through the agencies of proper staffing levels, effective supervision and monitoring, controlled, regulated progression into role demands and in this process ensuring a curriculum that meets their needs and the needs of their patients in the immediate and long term.

Failure to address and remedy the deficiencies evidenced by nurses themselves will only serve to endorse the findings of Hunt (1992), who stated:

> There has always been a glaring discrepancy between the ideals of nursing and the realities of nursing practice with all its constraints. If the nursing profession as a whole remains unaware of the character and significance of current developments (and non-developments) in the health care delivery system it will continue to stand by and observe powerlessly as that discrepancy takes yet another new form, indeed a deeper and more pernicious form than ever.
>
> *(Para. 2, p. 91)*

A proposed vehicle for the realization of ideas inherent in the proposals already outlined could be addressed by enveloping preregistration and postregistration professional educational development of the nurse as a continuum, using as a framework the 'spiral curriculum'.

The spiral curriculum proposed engages the ideas of Bruner (1977) and Warwick (1987, 1988). In this respect, Bruner makes the following observations, central to which is the theme of the spiral curriculum: 'Learning should not only take us somewhere; it should allow us later to go further more easily' (para. 1, p. 17). Bruner's ideas comprise four themes including: 'The continued broadening and deepening of knowledge in terms of basic and general ideas; the role of structure in learning and how it may be made central in teaching; readiness for learning; the nature of intuition, the desire to learn and how it may be stimulated' (para. 2, pp. 11/12/13/14).

Warwick, in his explanation of the modular curriculum, defines 'module' as 'A single unit, complete in itself, but which may be added to further units towards the achievement of a larger task or a more long-term goal' (para. 1, p. 4). The modular curriculum described by Warwick is seen by him to have a number of advantages, which include the effects on student motivation because of the immediacy of the goal, the relatively easy plotting of an individual's progress and the provision of a test-bed for curricular innovation.

I propose combining the ideas of Bruner and Warwick into a composite educational framework. The synergistic approach thus created links together a modular and spiral approach to the curriculum. The proposed framework if thoughtfully designed, developed, monitored and evaluated could provide an effective educational framework by enhancing the linear, progressive and interdependent key components of the nursing curriculum at preregistration and postregistration levels, while simultaneously addressing specifically defined educational needs of nurses in their lifelong professional development.

The proposed framework (Fig. 2) is based on a spiral approach to nurses' development with the inherent philosophy of a concentric, ongoing develop-ment that addresses the educational and professional needs of nurses at different levels of the profession by progressing from the basic to the more advanced concepts, skills and knowledge. It also returns to basic concepts, skills and knowledge as professional or clinical needs dictate, simultaneously broadening, deepening, clarifying, extending and rebuilding them.

This gradual extending spiral to be effective in meeting nurses' needs must embody regular and continuous support, evaluation, performance appraisal and feedback and in this way encourage and enable the full use of their potential. Most importantly, the proposed curriculum must acknowledge nurses as persons with fears and anxieties as well as needs, which must be met in an ever-changing, demanding and complex role.

Central to the curricular philosophy is the provision of time for nurses' reflective thinking and the use of an action-learning approach to enable nurses to discuss their work-related problems and learn from each other in a climate of mutual understanding and trust.

The substance of the framework (education matter) is embodied in, and enhanced by, dynamic and realistic modules that meet nurses' needs fully and effectively, at different phases in their professional development. The proposed approach perceives nurses' development as a continuum that embodies logical, rational and progressive links and development, starting at the point of entry to the profession as a nursing student, ensuring a thorough grasp of the basic concepts and competencies of nursing theory and practice. This must be activated by practical experience in a controlled clinical environment where the needs of nursing students and their motivation are encouraged.

The approach is based on the reality of the demands on nurses throughout different phases of their professional career development and not on the ideal, unrealistic and unattainable. The scenario thus outlined envisages the nurse as having freedom to question practices without fear of reprimand or being made to feel uncomfortable, as this stunts the enrichment of nurses' intellectual and emotional development by not encouraging their creative and innovative ideas.

In the situation described, nurses would move smoothly and with confidence by preparation into the many different roles they undertake at preregistration and postregistration levels, thus reducing/obviating what Kramer (1974) referred to as 'reality shock', and its consequent disillusionment, apathy and stress. This approach envisages as a prerequisite to its efficacy the careful identification, definition, clarification, deepening and extension of the basic competencies and associated theory in the context of the skills, knowledge and expertise which progressively in the course of their career nurses are expected to address. Inherent in this framework are mini-spirals which depict the more profound, advanced and specialized periods in nurses' lifelong development.

Imperative in the effective use of this framework are Bruner's (1977) ideas: 'Subjects taught should have relevance, i.e. they are worth knowing; concepts should be encountered in a variety of contexts over a period of time and gradually assimilated rather than suddenly learned; learning experiences should be so arranged that the person works through the basic concepts of a subject before spiralling upwards; and tackle the same concepts again but at successively, more rigorous and sophisticated levels' (para. 2, p. 18).

The approach thus outlined, as well as embodying the ideas of acknowledged educationists and discussions with Warwick, was also influenced by the perceptions of the researcher, based on many years' experience in nurse education together with the perceptions of nurses taking part in the study, as to its usefulness in furthering staff development. The importance and value of the proposed framework lies in its flexibility, including its expandability and contractability enabling the prompt and appropriate addressing and accommodation of specific, desired educational outcomes, at any stage in nurses' development. It must be borne in mind that this framework does not attempt to prescribe content, but merely constitutes a vehicle in which nurses' educational needs are appropriately met.

The financial implications of the proper professional development of nurses in the light of the foregoing analysis makes economic good sense. Indeed, in light of current economic stringencies, the proposals for the development of nurses if taken seriously are many, great and ultimately cost-effective, and equate with having a workforce that is ready, confident, trained and prepared for each aspect of change and its consequent demands (see UKCC, 1987).

Finally, the nursing profession – nursing and health care in general – is confronted with major and wide-ranging change, possibly the most radical change in the history of the profession. Professionals must recognize and acknowledge the impediments that still plague it and realize that there is still much pessimism amongst staff which must be addressed before the profession can look optimistically at the overall effect of all the new initiatives. This pessimism must not be allowed to smoulder as it has in the past and jeopardize progressive developments. The profession must unite itself and take heed of past failures and missed opportunities and support the present initiatives. The profession has been given an opportunity to take itself with professional integrity, confidence and security into the next century, and it cannot afford to fail!

APPENDIX A

Confidential

_____

OBS WSCN SN

_____

A. GENERAL INFORMATION

Computer use

Date of study:

| 1 |

Time of study   Start: Finish:

Category of staff observed:

   1. Ward sister/charge nurse

   2. Staff nurse

1.

| | 1 |
| 2 |

Nature of sample/time: Rated $1\frac{1}{2}$ minute set intervals $\times 2$ hours/person

Ward profile

Nature of ward:

   1. Acute medical

   2. Acute surgical

   3. Longstay (geriatric)

3.

| | 1 |
| 2 |
| 3 |

Mix of patients:

   1. High dependency (maximum care)   5.

   2. Intermediate dependency (average care)

   3. Low dependency (virtual self-care)

	1
	2
	3

Ward membership:

   1. Male   7.

   2. Female

   3. Male and female

	1
	2
	3

District Health Authority: 9. [1]

Hospital: 11. [1]

Ward: 13. [1]

Non-participant observation schedule number   15. [1]

Role of nurse at time of observation:

   1. In charge of ward   17.

   2. Senior nurse (staff nurse)

	1
	2

Description of ward at time of observation:

B. STAFF ESTABLISHMENT

Staff establishment for ward (F.T.E. for each grade):

1. Ward sister/charge nurse	19.		1
2. Staff nurse			2
3. Enrolled nurse			3
4. Nursing students (if not supernumerary)			4
5. Care assistants (nursing auxiliaries)			5
6. Clerical assistants			6

Staff on duty at time of observation:

1. Ward sister/charge nurse	31.		1
2. Staff nurse			2
3. Enrolled nurse			3
4. Nursing students (if not supernumerary)			4
5. Care assistants (nursing auxiliaries)			5
6. Clerical assistants			6

1. Male	43.		1
2. Female			2

C. OPERATIONAL DEFINITIONS OF ROLE ACTIVITY ELEMENTS

The following operational definitions are used:
1. *Managerial:* Any activity which relates to the general management of the ward
2. *Administrative:* Any activity which relates to ward routine but **not** to patients' condition and/or care
3. *Clinical:* Any activity which relates to patients' condition (management of care), including time spent on direct care
4. *Education:* Any activity which relates to:
   (a) Formal teaching/instruction of nurses
   (b) Formally informing patients on matters relating to their health (health education), and care
5. *Communication:* Any activity which, in the context of this study relates to

the **direct** giving and receiving of information between the role occupant and:

(a) Nurses (directions, reports, discussion, or informal conversation)

(b) Doctors

(c) Patients

6. *Waiting:* Inactivity between tasks
7. *Resting:* Agreed/approved rest breaks
8. *Walking:* To and from station/office/activity
9. *Direct supervision of nurses:* Direct overseeing of nurses in the performance of clinical and/or managerial tasks
10. *Time on telephone:* Giving and receiving (G/R) varied information in relation to the ward management, the patients and ward nursing staff; also includes clarification of situations requested by nurse
11. *Macro elements:* Activity elicited through discussion with nurses, information presented in job-descriptions of the nurse and/or defined by the pre-pilot and pilot studies (not minutiae)
12. *Miscellaneous:* Any activity which is extra to elements 1–13

In addition to the sampling of the above elements, the observer will attempt to assess:

13. *Authority/power:* The degree of freedom of the role occupant to influence the behaviour of the ward team
14. *Autonomy:* The freedom of the role occupant to use their professional judgement
15. *High dependency patients:* Maximum care; the patient is totally dependent upon the nursing staff for his care.
16. *Intermediate dependency patients:* Average care; the patient is able to provide some care without assistance
17. *Low dependency patients:* Virtual self-care; the patient is quite independent for his personal care
18. *Duties/functions:* The tasks which are associated with the job of the trained nurse (deemed to be appropriate to role, by senior nursing management)
19. *Responsibilities:* Charges for which the nurse is answerable (deemed to be appropriate to role by the UKCC and senior nursing management)

D. ACTIVITY

Code: 1 = activity (behaviour) observed

	1	2	3	Education		Communication			Time On Tel. G.1 R.1	Dir. sup. of nurs.			
				4	5	6	7	8	9	10	11	12	13	14
Time: fixed time interval (1½ mins)	Mana-gerial	Admin.	Clinical	Nurses	Patients	Nurses	Doctors	Patients			Waiting	Resting	Walking	Misc.
Total														

Column/activity (macro elements)

E. ADDITIONAL INFORMATION

Direct quotations by nurse about job:

Skills in common use at time of observation:

Range of duties observed:

Range of responsibilities observed:

Miscellaneous activities:

Observer's reactions and reflections about what has occurred
  1. The ward environment:

  2. Interactions:

3. Own feelings (about what took place):

4. Summary:

APPENDIX B

JOB DESCRIPTIONS

NB. It was found that none of the job descriptions had been updated since the appointment of the post holder.

District Health Authority 1

A STANDARD GUIDE TO THE RESPONSIBILITIES AND THE ROLE OF THE SISTER/CHARGE NURSE (GRADE 6)

Location: Medical Unit.

Responsible to: The Sister/Charge Nurse is immediately responsible to the Clinical Services Manager and through the Clinical Services Manager to the Patient Services Manager for the duties and responsibilities of the post and other such duties as might be delegated by the Clinical Services Manager.

1 Summary of duties

The Sister/Charge Nurse is responsible to the Clinical Services Manager for the nursing service to the patients and for the control, training and well-being of the nursing staff in the Unit.

2 Duties and responsibilities

2.1 *Patient care*

     2.1.1   Responsible for the nursing care and welfare of all patients in the Unit, ensuring a high standard of nursing care by carrying out correct procedures.

2.1.2   Allocation and supervision of work to nursing staff, ensuring they are continuously aware of the condition of the patients.

2.1.3   Supervising treatments ordered by medical staff and ensuring that nursing staff are aware of treatment regimes ordered.

2.1.4   Keeping the Clinical Services Manager and medical staff informed of patients' treatments and progress.

2.1.5   Keeping full and accurate nursing records.

2.1.6   Reporting untoward incidents in accordance with the agreed procedures

2.1.7   Maintaining custody of controlled drugs and other drugs in accordance with the rules laid down in the standard procedures and legal requirements and ensuring the correct administration and recording of drugs and medication.

2.1.8   Informing patients' relatives of the progress and condition of the patients.

2.1.9   Co-operating with all wards in the hospital, especially those which patients are transferred to or from.

2.1.10 Co-operating with staff from other wards and those concerned with other services to the patients.

2.2 *Nurse training*

2.2.1   Be aware of the aims and objectives of the Student Nurses in the medical allocation.

2.2.2   Be an assessor for ward-based examinations for learners.

2.2.3   Be prepared to undertake a Clinical Teaching Course.

2.2.4   Prepare, carry out, review and revise programmes of training in nursing techniques and ward management for all grades of nursing staff in the ward in consultation with the Clinical Services Manager.

2.2.5   Carry out a regular programme of training for all grades of nursing staff, as agreed with the Clinical Services Manager.

2.2.6   Participate in study days and courses for nursing staff below the grade of Sister/Charge Nurse, when required.

2.2.7   Co-operate with the Nursing Officer, In-Service Training and the Nurse Teaching Centre.

2.3 *General co-ordination*

2.3.1   Return information on patients as required by the Clinical Services Manager.

2.3.2   Ensure all equipment, furnishings and accommodation are adequately maintained in good order and are properly used. Report defects to the correct department.

2.3.3   Ensure that adequate supplies of all relevant requirements are provided, having due regard to economy.

2.3.4   Attend meetings arranged by the Clinical Services Manager to discuss problems and exchange views and ideas for the improvement of services provided.

2.3.5   Establish and maintain good working relationships with all disciplines within South West Durham Health Authority.

2.3.6   Attend fire lectures and ensure that all staff within the section are aware of fire precautions, knowing the location of fire-fighting equipment and how to use same.

All nursing staff are expected to keep abreast of current trends of development in medical and nursing practice. The Sister/Charge Nurse will be expected to attend and participate in relevant conferences, courses and study days.

It is expected that all nursing staff will be available for day or night duty as the Service needs arise to further clinical experience and career development, as the opportunity occurs.

This Job Description indicates the main functions and responsibilities of the post. It is not intended to be a complete list and, in agreement with the holder of the post, will be amended, as necessary, in the event of future change or experience.

31.7.86

A STANDARD GUIDE TO THE RESPONSIBILITIES AND THE ROLE OF THE SISTER/CHARGE NURSE (GRADE 6)

Location: Surgical Unit.

Responsible to: The Sister/Charge Nurse is immediately responsible to the Clinical Services Manager and through the Clinical Services Manager to the Patient Services Manager for the duties and responsibilities of the post and other such duties as might be delegated by the Clinical Services Manager.

1 Summary of duties

The Sister/Charge Nurse is responsible to the Clinical Services Manager for the nursing service to the patients and for the control, training and well-being of the nursing staff in the Unit.

2 Duties and responsibilities

2.1 *Patient care*

2.1.1   Responsible for the nursing care and welfare of all patients in the Unit, ensuring a high standard of nursing care by carrying out correct procedures.

2.1.2   Allocation and supervision of work to nursing staff, ensuring they are continuously aware of the condition of the patients.

2.1.3   Supervising treatments ordered by medical staff and ensuring that nursing staff are aware of treatment regimes ordered.

2.1.4   Keeping the Clinical Services Manager and medical staff informed of patients' treatments and progress.

2.1.5   Keeping full and accurate nursing records.

2.1.6   Reporting untoward incidents in accordance with the agreed procedures.

2.1.7   Maintaining custody of controlled drugs and other drugs in accordance with the rules laid down in the standard procedures and legal requirements and ensuring the correct administration and recording of drugs and medication.

2.1.8   Informing patients' relatives of the progress and condition of the patients.

2.1.9   Co-operating with all wards in the hospital, especially those which patients are transferred to or from.

2.1.10 Co-operating with staff from other wards and those concerned with other services to the patients.

2.2 *Nurse training*

2.2.1   Be aware of the aims and objectives of the Student Nurses in the medical allocation.

2.2.2   Be an assessor for ward-based examinations for learners.

2.2.3   Be prepared to undertake a Clinical Teaching Course.

2.2.4   Prepare, carry out, review and revise programmes of training in nursing techniques and ward management for all grades of nursing staff in the ward in consultation with the Clinical Services Manager.

2.2.5   Carry out a regular programme of training for all grades of nursing staff, as agreed with the Clinical Services Manager.

2.2.6   Participate in study days and courses for nursing staff below the grade of Sister/Charge Nurse, when required.

2.2.7   Co-operate with the Nursing Officer, In-Service Training and the Nurse Teaching Centre.

2.3 *General co-ordination*

2.3.1   Return information on patients as required by the Clinical
Services Manager.

2.3.2   Ensure all equipment, furnishing and accommodation are
adequately maintained in good order and are properly used.
Report defects to the correct department.

2.3.3   Ensure that adequate supplies of all relevant requirements are
provided, having due regard to economy.

2.3.4   Attend meetings arranged by the Clinical Services Manager to
discuss problems and exchange views and ideas for the
improvement of services provided.

2.3.5   Establish and maintain good working relationships with all
disciplines within South West Durham Health Authority.

2.3.6.   Attend fire lectures and ensure that all staff within the section
are aware of fire precautions, knowing the location of fire-
fighting equipment and how to use same.

All nursing staff are expected to keep abreast of current trends of development
in medical and nursing practice. The Sister/Charge Nurse will be expected to
attend and participate in relevant conferences, courses and study days.

**It is expected that all nursing staff will be available for day or night duty as the
Service needs arise to further clinical experience and career development, as the
opportunity occurs.**

This Job Description indicates the main functions and responsibilities of the
post. It is not intended to be a complete list and, in agreement with the holder
of the post, will be amended, as necessary, in the event of future change or
experience.

31.7.86

**A GUIDE TO THE RESPONSIBILITIES OF THE SISTER/CHARGE
NURSE IN CHARGE (GRADE 6) ACUTE GERIATRIC UNIT AND
DAY HOSPITAL**

Responsible to: The Sister/Charge Nurse will be responsible to the Unit
Nursing Officer and through her to the Divisional
Nursing Officer for the day-to-day management of the
unit. The Nursing Officer will be available to support.

Duties and responsibilities

1 *Patient care*

   (a) Entirely responsible for a high standard of nursing care and for the welfare of all patients and development of the Nursing Process.
   (b) Ensuring that correct procedures are carried out by **all** grades of nursing staff by constant observation and supervision.
   (c) Ensuring that nursing staff are aware of treatments ordered and discontinued by medical staff and that account is taken of this when Nursing Profiles and Care Plans are prepared.
   (d) Keeping medical staff and Nursing Officer informed of patients' progress.
   (e) Allocating and supervising the work of the nursing staff.
   (f) Maintaining continuous contact with the patients to observe their progress and ensure their comfort and care.
   (g) Maintaining the custody of dangerous drugs and poisons in accordance with the rules laid down.
   (h) Co-operating with staff of other services to the patient.
   (i) Communicating with patients' relatives on all matters concerning the patients' welfare.
   (j) Reporting to medical staff and Nursing Officer any untoward incident regarding the patients.
   (k) Responsible for staff seconded from other departments.

2 *Nursing staff*

   (a) Responsible for the control, training and well-being of the nursing staff.
   (b) Reviewing and revising programmes of training in nursing techniques and management for all grades of staff.
   (c) If qualified, acting as an examiner for assessment of nurses when required.
   (d) Participating in study days and courses for nursing staff below the grade of Sister/Charge Nurse when required.

3 *General co-ordination*

   (a) Responsible for the organization of nursing staff allocated and to provide adequate coverage at all times and informing the Nursing Officer when this is not possible.
   (b) Returning information on patients and staff as requested by the Nursing Officer.
   (c) Co-operating with Domestic Superintendent and Catering Officer in order to obtain the best possible service to the patients.

(d) Ensuring that **adequate** supplies are provided and discourage **borrowing** from other wards and departments as far as possible.

(e) Ensuring all equipment is kept well maintained and ready for use and that all grades of nursing staff are aware of the location of such equipment.

(f) Attend monthly meetings convened by Nursing Officer.

(g) 'Acting up' for Nursing Officer when required.

(h) Co-operate with Control of Infection Officers (medical and nursing).

(i) Assist Sector Administrator in the welfare and safety of both staff and patients especially with regard to fire precautions.

(j) Establish and maintain good working relationships with Sector Administrator and heads of departments.

(k) Co-operate fully with night Sisters and Nursing Officer responsible for night supervision.

(l) Providing information for Nursing Officer when accidents and incidents involving patients and staff are being investigated.

(m) Providing information for Nursing Officer when complaints against Nursing Services are being investigated.

All Nursing Staff are expected to keep abreast of current trends and developments in medical and nursing practice. Job holders will be expected to attend and participate in relevant conferences, courses, etc. It is expected that all nursing staff will be available for day/night duty as the service need arises to further career development and to further clinical experience as the opportunity arises.

This job description indicates the main functions and responsibilities of the post. It is not intended to be a complete list and, in agreement with the job holder, will be amended as necessary in the event of future change or experience.

8.7.81

A STANDARD GUIDE TO THE RESPONSIBILITIES AND THE ROLE OF THE STAFF NURSE

Responsible to: The Staff Nurse will be responsible to the Ward Sister and to the Clinical Services Manager, and through him/her to the Patient Services Manager for the day-to-day management of the ward, in Sister/Charge Nurse's absence. The Clinical Services Manager will be available to support, advise or assist the ward or unit staff – particularly the Staff Nurse to whom the Sister/Charge Nurse has delegated his/her responsibilities.

Duties and responsibilities

Patient care

1. Entirely responsible for a high standard of nursing care and for the welfare of all patients on the ward.
2. Ensuring that correct procedures are carried out by **all** grades of nursing staff, by constant observation and supervision.
3. Ensuring that nursing staff are aware of treatments ordered and discontinued by medical staff.
4. Keeping medical staff and Clinical Services Manager informed of patients' progress.
5. Allocating and supervising the work of the nursing staff.
6. Maintaining continuous contact with the patients to observe their progress and ensure their comfort and care.
7. Maintaining the custody of dangerous drugs and poisons in accordance with the rules laid down by the Health Authority and ensuring the checking and administration of drugs and poisons.
8. Co-operation with staff of other services to the patient.
9. Communicating with patients' relatives on all matters concerning the patients' welfare.
10. Reporting to medical staff and Clinical Service Manager any untoward incident regarding the patients.
11. Responsible for staff seconded to sections from other departments.

Nursing staff

1. Responsible for the control, training and well-being of the nursing staff in the ward or section.
2. Responsible for all communications at ward level.

General co-ordination

1. Returning information on patients, as requested by the Clinical Services Manager.
2. Returning information about staff, as requested by the Clinical Services Manager.
3. Co-operation with Domestic Services Manager and Catering Manager in order to obtain the best possible service to the ward and patients.
4. Ensuring that **adequate** stocks of supplies are provided and discourage **borrowing** from other wards and departments as far as possible.
5. Ensuring all equipment is kept well maintained and ready for use and that all grades of nursing staff are aware of the location of such equipment.
6. Assist hospital administration in the welfare and safety of both staff and patients, especially with regard to fire precautions.

7. Establish and maintain good working relationships with Support Services Manager and Heads of Departments.
8. Co-operate fully with the Clinical Services Managers and Night Sisters responsible for night supervision.
9. Providing information for Clinical Services Managers when accidents and incidents involving patients and staff are being investigated.
10. Providing information to Clinical Services Manager when complaints against the nursing service are being investigated.

This guide is not intended as a complete list of duties and responsibilities but indicates the important needs of the post. The understanding and appreciation of the role of first line managers is essential as is consultation with and the co-operation of all the professions and disciplines involved, either directly or indirectly in the provision of **patient care**.

It may be necessary to amend this guide from time to time in the future, in order to take into account the changing pattern of nurse training and patient care.

All nursing staff are expected to keep abreast of current trends and developments in medical and nursing practice, and be prepared to receive training and become proficient in other procedures which are not part of a nurse's normal role.

It is expected that all nursing staff will be available for day/night duty as the service need arises to further career development and to further clinical experience as the opportunity arises.

April 1988

District Health Authority 2

A GUIDE TO THE JOB OF THE NURSING SISTER/CHARGE NURSE

Job title: Nursing Sister/Charge Nurse

Position in organization:
(a) Directly responsible to Unit Nursing Officer.
(b) Subordinates directly supervised: Staff Nurses
State Enrolled Nurses
Student Nurses
Pupil Nurses
Nursing Auxiliaries
Domestic Staff (sapiential authority)

Main purpose of job:
1. To control the ward, department or attachment and organize the work in order to provide high standards of patient care.
2. To maintain the safety of patients and staff.
3. To pass on nursing skills and teach the learners.

Main personal activities:
1. Supervision of patient care.
2. Direction of subordinate staff.
3. Communicating Nursing and Management Policies to Junior Medical Staff and subordinate staff, and providing feedback to Unit Nursing Officer.

Nursing Sister/Charge Nurse: His/her responsibilities

Responsibility to Patient and his relatives	—safety —well-being —high standards of care
Responsibility to Medical Staff	—carrying out of medical instructions —safety —communications
Responsibility to Learners	—teaching —passing on of skills —counselling
Responsibility to Organization	—safety —control —communications —personal contribution
Responsibility to Profession	—communication —personal contribution —personnel development
Responsibility to Oneself	—current awareness —personal development

A detailed definition of these responsibilities **and of the standard expected** in each of the areas identified will be given to you if you are successful in obtaining an appointment. This will form the basis for assessment of progress on the job.

1 November 1979

A GUIDE TO THE JOB OF STAFF NURSE/MIDWIFE

Job title: Staff Nurse/Midwife

Position in organization:
(a) Directly responsible to Ward Sister/Charge Nurse
(b) Subordinates directly supervised: State Enrolled Nurses
                                        Student Nurses
                                        Pupil Nurses
                                        Nursing Auxiliaries
                                        Domestic Staff (sapiential authority)

Main purpose of job:
1. To lead a team and give support to other staff to enable nursing care plans to be carried through.
2. To control the ward, department or attachment and organize the work in order to provide high standards of patient care in the absence of Sister.
3. To maintain the safety of patients and staff.
4. To pass on nursing skills and teach the learners.

Main personal activities
1. Supervision and participation in patient care.
2. Direction and organization of subordinate staff.
3. Understanding and communicating Nursing and Management Policies to medical staff and subordinate staff, and providing feedback to Sister.

Staff Nurse/Midwife: His/her responsibilities

Responsibility to Patient (and his relatives)	—safety —well-being —high standards of care
Responsibility to Medical Staff	—carrying out of orders (reliability) —safety —communications
Responsibility to Learners	—teaching —passing on of skills —counselling
Responsibility to Organization	—safety —control —communications —personal contribution
Responsibility to Profession	—communication —personal contribution —personal development

Responsibility to Oneself —current awareness
—personal development

A detailed definition of these responsibilities **and of the standard expected** in each of the areas identified will be given to you if you are successful in obtaining an appointment. This will form the basis for assessment of progress on the job.

November 1979

APPENDIX C

**RATING BY OTHER PROFESSIONALS OF THE EXTENT NURSES'
PRESCRIBED DUTIES FEATURED IN THEIR JOB**

UNIT NURSE MANAGERS

Clinical (management of patient care) ($n = 6$)

Q. The following is a list of duties assumed to be appropriate by Senior Nurse
Management to the role of the professional nurse. Indicate to what extent
you perceive they feature in their job.

	Great extent	Fair extent	Some extent	Little extent
1. Determining nursing policy	16.66	–	66.66	16.66
2. Identifying patients' needs	83.33	16.66	–	–
3. Prescribing nurses' work (in the context of nursing care and medical instructions)	83.33	–	16.66	–
4. Planning nursing care (defining patient-care objectives)	83.33	–	16.66	–
5. Delivering nursing care (having direct contact with patients)	–	83.33	16.66	–
6. Integrating the work of the ward team	66.66	16.66	16.66	–
7. Setting nursing standards (ensuring high standards of care)	83.33	–	16.66	–
8. Evaluating nursing care (against defined nursing objectives)	66.66	16.66	–	16.66

	Great extent	Fair extent	Some extent	Little extent
9. Fulfilling nurses' legal obligations (drugs, treatment)	100	–	–	–
10. Fulfilling nurses' ethical obligations to patients (confidentiality)	100	–	–	–
11. Ensuring the independence of patients (ensuring freedom of activity within prescribed levels)	33.33	50	16.66	–
12. Other	–	–	–	–

Managerial (general management of ward)

	Great extent	Fair extent	Some extent	Little extent
1. Deciding what work has to be done (establishing goals)	83.33	–	16.66	–
2. Allocating work	83.33	–	16.66	–
3. Co-ordinating the work of the ward team	66.66	16.66	16.66	–
4. Ensuring accountability for work done	66.66	16.66	16.66	–
5. Monitoring the work of nurses	83.33	–	16.66	–
6. Ensuring the adequacy of resources	33.33	–	50	16.66
7. Organizing resources (Matching resources to workload)	33.33	16.66	33.33	16.66
8. Communicating with ward team	83.33	–	16.66	–
9. Communicating with patients	83.33	16.66	–	–
10. Counselling staff	66.66	–	16.66	16.66
11. Appraising staff	66.66	16.66	–	16.66
12. Leading ward team	83.33	16.66	–	–

Administrative (ward routine but not patients' condition)

	Great extent	Fair extent	Some extent	Little extent
1. Ordering ward stock	33.33	16.66	16.66	16.66
2. Checking ward stock	33.33	–	16.66	–
3. Requisitioning resources	33.33	33.33	33.33	–
4. Preparing returns for nursing/hospital management	83.33	16.66	–	–
5. Writing reports	83.33	–	16.66	–
6. Arranging meetings (ward policy)	16.66	–	16.66	16.66

Educational (teaching, instructing and/or informing)

	Great extent	Fair extent	Some extent	Little extent
1. Induction of trained nurses (new to ward)	83.33	–	–	1, NR
2. Induction of nursing students (new to ward)	50	33.33	–	1, NR
3. Planning the educational experience of nursing students	33.33	33.33	–	1, NR
4. Teaching staff	83.33	16.66	–	–
5. Teaching patients (health education)	66.66	16.66	–	1, NR
6. Counsel staff as appropriate	50	33.33	–	1, NR

SENIOR NURSE MANAGERS

Clinical (management of patient care) ($n = 2$)

Q. The following is a list of duties assumed to be appropriate by Senior Nurse Management to the role of the professional nurse. Indicate to what extent you perceive they feature in their job.

	Great extent	Fair extent	Some extent	Little extent
1. Determining nursing policy	–	–	50	50
2. Identifying patients' needs	–	100	–	–
3. Prescribing nurses' work (in the context of nursing care and medical instructions)	50	50	–	–
4. Planning nursing care (defining patient-care objectives)	100	–	–	–
5. Delivering nursing care (having direct contact with patients)	50	50	–	–
6. Integrating the work of the ward team	100	–	–	–
7. Setting nursing standards (ensuring high standards of care)	50	50	–	–
8. Evaluating nursing care (against defined nursing objectives)	100	–	–	–
9. Fulfilling nurses' legal obligations (drugs, treatment)	100	–	–	–
10. Fulfilling nurses' ethical obligations to patients (confidentiality)	100	–	–	–
11. Ensuring the independence of patients (ensuring freedom of activity within prescribed levels)	–	100	–	–
12. Other	–	–	–	–

Managerial (general management of ward)

	Great extent	Fair extent	Some extent	Little extent
1. Deciding what work has to be done (establishing goals)	50	50	–	–
2. Allocating work	–	100	–	–
3. Co-ordinating the work of the ward team	50	50	–	–
4. Ensuring accountability for work done	–	100	–	–
5. Monitoring the work of nurses	–	100	–	–
6. Ensuring the adequacy of resources	50	–	50	–
7. Organizing resources (matching resources to workload)	–	–	100	–
8. Communicating with ward team	100	–	–	–
9. Communicating with patients	100	–	–	–
10. Counselling staff	–	50	50	–
11. Appraising staff	–	100	–	–
12. Leading ward team	100	–	–	–

Administrative (ward routine but not patients' condition)

	Great extent	Fair extent	Some extent	Little extent
1. Ordering ward stock	–	50	50	–
2. Checking ward stock	–	50	50	–
3. Requisitioning resources	–	100	–	–
4. Preparing returns for nursing/hospital management	–	100	–	–
5. Writing reports	–	100	–	–
6. Arranging meetings (ward policy)	–	50	50	–

Educational (teaching, instructing and/or informing)

	Great extent	Fair extent	Some extent	Little extent
1. Induction of trained nurses (new to ward)	50	50	–	–
2. Induction of nursing students (new to ward)	50	50	–	–
3. Planning the educational experience of nursing students	100	–	–	–
4. Teaching staff	–	50	50	–
5. Teaching patients (health education)	–	50	50	–
6. Counsel staff as appropriate	–	100	–	–

DOCTORS

Clinical (management of patient care) ($n = 29$)

Q. The following is a list of duties assumed to be appropriate by Senior Nurse Management to the role of the professional nurse. Indicate to what extent you perceive they feature in their job.

	Great extent	Fair extent	Some extent	Little extent
1. Determining nursing policy	13.79	31.03	24.13	31.03
2. Identifying patients' needs	58.62	27.58	13.79	–
3. Prescribing nurses' work (in the context of nursing care and medical instructions)	48.22	48.27	3.44	–
4. Planning nursing care (defining patient-care objectives)	44.82	48.27	6.89	–
5. Delivering nursing care (having direct contact with patients)	44.82	20.68	24.13	10.34
6. Integrating the work of the ward team	17.24	58.63	20.68	3.44

	Great extent	Fair extent	Some extent	Little extent
7. Setting nursing standards (ensuring high standards of care)	27.58	58.62	13.79	–
8. Evaluating nursing care (against defined nursing objectives)	20.68	24.13	24.13	31.03
9. Fulfilling nurses' legal obligations (drugs, treatment)	75.86	13.79	6.89	1, NR
10. Fulfilling nurses' ethical obligations to patients (confidentiality)	75.86	13.79	6.89	1, NR
11. Ensuring the independence of patients (ensuring freedom of activity within prescribed levels)	31.03	57.72	17.24	–
12. Other	–	–	–	–

Managerial (general management of ward)

	Great extent	Fair extent	Some extent	Little extent
1. Deciding what work has to be done (establishing goals)	51.72	44.82	–	1, NR
2. Allocating work	62.06	27.58	6.89	3.44
3. Co-ordinating the work of the ward team	31.03	44.82	24.13	–
4. Ensuring accountability for work done	17.24	41.37	31.03	10.34
5. Monitoring the work of nurses	24.13	31.03	34.48	10.34
6. Ensuring the adequacy of resources	10.34	10.34	13.79	65.51
7. Organizing resources (matching resources to workload)	17.24	17.24	17.24	48.27
8. Communicating with ward team	48.27	44.82	3.44	3.44

	Great extent	Fair extent	Some extent	Little extent
9. Communicating with patients	51.72	31.03	17.24	–
10. Counselling staff	10.34	34.48	31.03	4, NR 10.34
11. Appraising staff	13.79	2, NR 31.03	37.93	2, NR 6.89
12. Leading ward team	37.93	27.58	17.24	17.24

Administrative (ward routine but not patients' condition)

	Great extent	Fair extent	Some extent	Little extent
1. Ordering ward stock	79.31	13.79	6.89	–
2. Checking ward stock	1, NR 65.51	24.13	6.89	–
3. Requisitioning resources	1, NR 65.51	24.13	6.89	–
4. Preparing returns for nursing/hospital management	79.31	20.68	–	–
5. Writing reports	89.65	3.44	6.89	–
6. Arranging meetings (ward policy)	17.24	6.89	24.13	5, NR 34.48

Educational (teaching, instructing and/or informing)

	Great extent	Fair extent	Some extent	Little extent
1. Induction of trained nurses (new to ward)	17.24	34.48	31.03	5, NR
2. Induction of nursing students (new to ward)	13.79	27.58	24.13	9, NR 3.44

	Great extent	Fair extent	Some extent	Little extent
3. Planning the educational experience of nursing students	6.89	13.79	31.03	8, NR 20.68
4. Teaching staff	10.34	13.79	41.37	3, NR 24.13
5. Teaching patients (health education)	13.79	31.03	37.93	20.68
6. Counsel staff as appropriate	13.79	13.79	34.48	5, NR 20.68

STATUTORY BODIES

Clinical (management of patient care) ($n = 2$)

Q. The following is a list of duties assumed to be appropriate by Senior Nurse Management to the role of the professional nurse. Indicate to what extent you perceive they feature in their job.

	Great extent	Fair extent	Some extent	Little extent
1. Determining nursing policy	–	–	100	–
2. Identifying patients' needs	–	100	–	–
3. Prescribing nurses' work (in the context of nursing care and medical instructions)	–	100	–	–
4. Planning nursing care (defining patient-care objectives)	–	–	50	50
5. Delivering nursing care (having direct contact with patients)	–	50	–	50
6. Integrating the work of the ward team	–	50	50	–
7. Setting nursing standards (ensuring high standards of care)	–	50	50	–
8. Evaluating nursing care (against defined nursing objectives)	–	–	50	50

	Great extent	Fair extent	Some extent	Little extent
9. Fulfilling nurses' legal obligations (drugs, treatment)	–	100	–	–
10. Fulfilling nurses' ethical obligations to patients (confidentiality)	–	50	–	50
11. Ensuring the independence of patients (ensuring freedom of activity within prescribed levels)	–	–	50	50
12. Other	–	–	–	–

Managerial (general management of ward)

	Great extent	Fair extent	Some extent	Little extent
1. Deciding what work has to be done (establishing goals)	–	100	–	–
2. Allocating work	–	100	–	–
3. Co-ordinating the work of the ward team	–	50	50	–
4. Ensuring accountability for work done	–	50	50	–
5. Monitoring the work of nurses	–	50	50	–
6. Ensuring the adequacy of resources	–	–	–	100
7. Organizing resources (matching resources to workload)	–	–	–	100
8. Communicating with ward team	–	50	–	50
9. Communicating with patients	–	50	–	50
10. Counselling staff	–	–	50	50
11. Appraising staff	–	50	50	–
12. Leading ward team	–	–	–	100

Administrative (ward routine but not patients' condition)

	Great extent	Fair extent	Some extent	Little extent
1. Ordering ward stock		No comment		
2. Checking ward stock		No comment		
3. Requisitioning resources		No comment		
4. Preparing returns for nursing/hospital management	100	–	–	–
5. Writing reports	100	–	–	–
6. Arranging meetings (ward policy)		No comment		

Educational (teaching, instructing and/or informing)

	Great extent	Fair extent	Some extent	Little extent
1. Induction of trained nurses (new to ward)		No comment		
2. Induction of nursing students (new to ward)		No comment		
3. Planning the educational experience of nursing students		No comment		
4. Teaching staff	–	–	–	–
5. Teaching patients (health education)	–	–	50	50
6. Counsel staff as appropriate	–	–	100	–

PROFESSIONAL BODY

Clinical (management of patient care) ($n = 1$)

Q. The following is a list of duties assumed to be appropriate by Senior Nurse Management to the role of the professional nurse. Indicate to what extent you perceive they feature in their job. ($\sqrt{}$ = response)

	Great extent	Fair extent	Some extent	Little extent
1. Determining nursing policy			$\sqrt{}$	
2. Identifying patients' needs	$\sqrt{}$			
3. Prescribing nurses' work (in the context of nursing care and medical instructions)	$\sqrt{}$			
4. Planning nursing care (defining patient-care objectives)			$\sqrt{}$	
5. Delivering nursing care (having direct contact with patients)		$\sqrt{}$		
6. Integrating the work of the ward team			$\sqrt{}$	
7. Setting nursing standards (ensuring high standards of care)			$\sqrt{}$	
8. Evaluating nursing care (against defined nursing objectives)				$\sqrt{}$
9. Fulfilling nurses' legal obligations (drugs, treatment)		$\sqrt{}$		
10. Fulfilling nurses' ethical obligations to patients (confidentiality)		$\sqrt{}$		
11. Ensuring the independence of patients (ensuring freedom of activity within prescribed levels)			$\sqrt{}$	
12. Other	–	–	–	–

Managerial (general management of ward)

	Great extent	Fair extent	Some extent	Little extent
1. Deciding what work has to be done (establishing goals)	√			
2. Allocating work	√			
3. Co-ordinating the work of the ward team		√		
4. Ensuring accountability for work done		√		
5. Monitoring the work of nurses		√		
6. Ensuring the adequacy of resources				√
7. Organizing resources (matching resources to workload)				√
8. Communicating with ward team		√		
9. Communicating with patients		√		
10. Counselling staff				√
11. Appraising staff			√	
12. Leading ward team				√

Administrative (ward routine but not patients' condition)

	Great extent	Fair extent	Some extent	Little extent
1. Ordering ward stock		√		
2. Checking ward stock		√		
3. Requisitioning resources		√		
4. Preparing returns for nursing/hospital management	√			

	Great extent	Fair extent	Some extent	Little extent
5. Writing reports	√			
6. Arranging meetings (ward policy)			√	

Education (teaching, instructing and/or informing)

	Great extent	Fair extent	Some extent	Little extent
1. Induction of trained nurses (new to ward)			√	
2. Induction of nursing students (new to ward)			√	
3. Planning the educational experience of nursing students			√	
4. Teaching staff				√
5. Teaching patients (health education)				√
6. Counsel staff as appropriate				√

APPENDIX D

RATING BY OTHER PROFESSIONALS OF THE NURSES' ABILITY TO MEET THEIR RESPONSIBILITIES

UNIT NURSE MANAGERS

Clinical

Q. The following is a list of responsibilities defined by the UKCC and Senior Nurse Management in relation to the job of the professional nurse. Indicate how far it is possible to meet these responsibilities in doing their job.

	Completely	To a reasonable degree	On the whole Yes	Not usually	Impossible
1. Act always to promote and safeguard the wellbeing of patients	50	50	–	–	–
2. Take account of the customs of patients	16.66	50	33.33	–	–
3. Carry out medical instructions	66.66	16.66	16.66	–	–
4. Ensure high standards of care	50	33.33	16.66	–	–
5. Respect the confidential information of patients	100	–	–	–	–
6. Ensure safe standards of practice (supervision of work)	–	66.66	33.33	–	–

	Completely	To a reasonable degree	On the whole Yes	Not usually	Impossible
7. Inform persons as appropriate of patient's progress (relatives, doctor, senior nursing manager)	66.66	33.33	–	–	–

Managerial

	Completely	To a reasonable degree	On the whole Yes	Not usually	Impossible
1. Work in a collaborative manner with other health-care professionals	50	33.33	16.66	–	–
2. Make known to an appropriate person/authority any conscientious objection relative to professional practice	83.33	16.66	–	–	–
3. Ensure the adequacy of resources	–	33.33	–	66.66	–
4. Make known to an appropriate person/authority circumstances which militate against safe standards of practice	50	16.66	33.33	–	–
5. Have regard to the workload on colleagues	33.33	16.66	33.33	16.66	–
6. Have regard to the workload on subordinates	33.33	16.66	33.33	16.66	–
7. Have regard to the pressures on colleagues	33.33	16.66	33.33	16.66	–

	Completely	To a reasonable degree	On the whole Yes	Not usually	Impossible
8. Have regard to the pressures on subordinates	33.33	33.33	16.66	16.66	–
9. Take action to reduce the workload on colleagues	16.66	33.33	16.66	33.33	–
10. Take action to reduce the workload on subordinates	16.66	33.33	16.66	33.33	–
11. Take action to reduce undue pressures on colleagues	16.66	33.33	16.66	33.33	–
12. Take action to reduce the pressures on subordinates	16.66	33.33	16.66	33.33	–

Educational

	Completely	To a reasonable degree	On the whole Yes	Not usually	Impossible
1. Improve own professional competence – skills and knowledge (specific)	50	16.66	16.66	16.66	–
2. Assist colleagues to develop professional competence (skills and knowledge)	50	50	–	–	–
3. Assist subordinates to develop professional competence (passing on of skills and knowledge)	50	33.33	16.66	–	–
4. Teach subordinates	50	16.66	33.33	–	–
5. Advise patients (health education)	66.66	33.33	–	–	–

	Completely	To a reasonable degree	On the whole Yes	Not usually	Impossible
6. Counsel staff as appropriate	50	33.33	–	16.66	–
7. Ensure own professional development (general)	33.33	33.33	33.33	–	–
8. Prepare programmes of training (nursing techniques and ward management)	50	16.66	–	16.66	1, NR
9. Act as assessor (ward-based examinations)	50	16.66	33.33	–	–

Educational

	Completely	To a reasonable degree	On the whole Yes	Not usually	Impossible
1. Improve own professional competence – skills and knowledge (specific)	50	16.66	16.66	16.66	–
2. Assist colleagues to develop professional competence (skills and knowledge)	50	50	–	–	–
3. Assist subordinates to develop professional competence (passing on of skills and knowledge)	50	33.33	16.66	–	–
4. Teach subordinates	50	16.66	33.33	–	–
5. Advise patients (health education)	66.66	33.33	–	–	–
6. Counsel staff as appropriate	50	33.33	–	16.66	–
7. Ensure own professional development (general)	33.33	33.33	33.33	–	–

	Completely	To a reasonable degree	On the whole Yes	Not usually	Impossible
8. Prepare programmes of training (nursing techniques and ward management)	50	16.66	–	16.66	1, NR
9. Act as assessor (ward-based examinations)	50	16.66	33.33	–	–

SENIOR NURSE MANAGERS

Clinical $(n=2)$

Q. The following is a list of responsibilities defined by the UKCC and Senior Nurse Management in relation to the job of the professional nurse. Indicate how far it is possible to meet these responsibilities in doing their job.

	Completely	To a reasonable degree	On the whole Yes	Not usually	Impossible
1. Act always to promote and safeguard the wellbeing of patients	50	–	50	–	–
2. Take account of the customs of patients	50	–	50	–	–
3. Carry out medical instructions	50	50	–	–	–
4. Ensure high standards of care	–	–	100	–	–
5. Respect the confidential information of patients	100	–	–	–	–
6. Ensure safe standards of practice (supervision of work)	–	50	50	–	–

	Completely	To a reasonable degree	On the whole Yes	Not usually	Impossible
7. Inform persons as appropriate of patient's progress (relatives, doctor, senior nursing manager)	50	50	–	–	–

Managerial

	Completely	To a reasonable degree	On the whole Yes	Not usually	Impossible
1. Work in a collaborative manner with other health-care professionals	–	100	–	–	–
2. Make known to an appropriate person/authority any conscientious objection relative to professional practice	50	–	50	–	–
3. Ensure the adequacy of resources	–	–	50	50	–
4. Make known to an appropriate person/authority circumstances which militate against safe standards of practice	–	–	100	–	–
5. Have regard to the workload on colleagues	–	–	100	–	–
6. Have regard to the workload on subordinates	–	–	100	–	–
7. Have regard to the pressures on colleagues	–	–	100	–	–

	Completely	To a reasonable degree	On the whole Yes	Not usually	Impossible
8. Have regard to the pressures on subordinates	–	–	100	–	–
9. Take action to reduce the workload on colleagues	–	–	100	–	–
10. Take action to reduce the workload on subordinates	–	–	100	–	–
11. Take action to reduce undue pressures on colleagues	–	–	100	–	–
12. Take action to reduce the pressures on subordinates	–	–	100	–	–

Educational

	Completely	To a reasonable degree	On the whole Yes	Not usually	Impossible
1. Improve own professional competence – skills and knowledge (specific)	–	100	–	–	–
2. Assist colleagues to develop professional competence (skills and knowledge)	–	100	–	–	–
3. Assist subordinates to develop professional competence (passing on of skills and knowledge)	50	50	–	–	–
4. Teach subordinates	–	–	–	–	–
5. Advise patients (health education)	–	50	50	–	–

	Completely	To a reasonable degree	On the whole Yes	Not usually	Impossible
6. Counsel staff as appropriate	–	50	–	50	–
7. Ensure own professional development (general)	–	100	–	–	–
8. Prepare programmes of training (nursing techniques and ward management)	–	100	–	–	–
9. Act as assessor (ward-based examinations)	–	100	–	–	–

DOCTORS

Clinical ($n = 29$)

Q. The following is a list of responsibilities defined by the UKCC and Senior Nurse Management in relation to the job of the professional nurse. Indicate how far it is possible to meet these responsibilities in doing their job.

	Completely	To a reasonable degree	On the whole Yes	Not usually	Impossible
1. Act always to promote and safeguard the wellbeing of patients	13.79	37.93	41.37	–	6.89
2. Take account of the customs of patients	–	44.82	41.37	13.79	–
3. Carry out medical instructions	37.93	37.93	24.13	–	–
4. Ensure high standards of care	6.89	31.03	55.17	6.89	–
5. Respect the confidential information of patients	37.93	37.93	20.68	3.44	–

	Completely	To a reasonable degree	On the whole Yes	Not usually	Impossible
6. Ensure safe standards of practice (supervision of work)	6.39	27.58	48.27	10.34	6.89
7. Inform persons as appropriate of patient's progress (relatives, doctor, senior nursing manager)	13.79	62.06	20.68	3.44	–

Managerial

	Completely	To a reasonable degree	On the whole Yes	Not usually	Impossible
1. Work in a collaborative manner with other health-care professionals	20.68	51.72	24.13	3.44	–
2. Make known to an appropriate person/authority any conscientious objection relative to professional practice	34.48	24.13	17.24	17.24	2, NR
3. Ensure the adequacy of resources	3.44	–	17.24	17.24	62.06
4. Make known to an appropriate person/authority circumstances which militate against safe standards of practice	13.79	17.24	58.62	6.89	6.89
5. Have regard to the workload on colleagues	–	17.24	34.48	10.34	37.94
6. Have regard to the workload on subordinates	–	10.34	41.37	13.79	34.50

	Completely	To a reasonable degree	On the whole Yes	Not usually	Impossible
7. Have regard to the pressures on colleagues	–	17.24	34.48	10.34	37.93
8. Have regard to the pressures on subordinates	–	10.34	41.39	13.79	34.48
9. Take action to reduce the workload on colleagues	–	3.44	10.34	17.26	68.96
10. Take action to reduce the workload on subordinates	–	3.44	10.34	20.71	65.51
11. Take action to reduce undue pressures on colleagues	–	3.44	10.34	17.24	65.51
12. Take action to reduce the pressures on subordinates	–	3.44	13.79	17.24	65.53

Educational

	Completely	To a reasonable degree	On the whole Yes	Not usually	Impossible
1. Improve own professional competence – skills and knowledge (specific)	–	6.89	48.27	34.48	3, NR
2. Assist colleagues to develop professional competence (skills and knowledge)	3.44	3.44	37.93	44.82	3, NR
3. Assist subordinates to develop professional competence (passing on of skills and knowledge)	3.44	13.79	41.37	31.03	3, NR
4. Teach subordinates	3.44	17.24	31.03	34.48	4, NR

	Completely	To a reasonable degree	On the whole Yes	Not usually	Impossible
5. Advise patients (health education)	–	10.34	41.37	41.37	6.89
6. Counsel staff as appropriate	–	6.89	31.03	37.93	7, NR
7. Ensure own professional development (general)	–	6.89	41.37	24.13	7, NR
8. Prepare programmes of training (nursing techniques and ward management)	–	10.34	24.13	24.13	3.44 11, NR
9. Act as assessor (ward-based examinations)	–	13.79	3.44	13.79	20, NR

STATUTORY BODIES

Clinical $(n = 2)$

Q. The following is a list of responsibilities defined by the UKCC and Senior Nurse Management in relation to the job of the professional nurse. Indicate how far it is possible to meet these responsibilities in doing their job.

	Completely	To a reasonable degree	On the whole Yes	Not usually	Impossible
1. Act always to promote and safeguard the wellbeing of patients	–	–	50	50	–
2. Take account of the customs of patients	–	–	100	–	–
3. Carry out medical instructions	50	50	–	–	–
4. Ensure high standards of care	–	–	50	50	–

	Completely	To a reasonable degree	On the whole Yes	Not usually	Impossible
5. Respect the confidential information of patients	–	100	–	–	–
6. Ensure safe standards of practice (supervision of work)	–	–	50	50	–
7. Inform persons as appropriate of patient's progress (relatives, doctor, senior nursing manager)	–	100	–	–	–

Managerial

	Completely	To a reasonable degree	On the whole Yes	Not usually	Impossible
1. Work in a collaborative manner with other health-care professionals	–	50	50	–	–
2. Make known to an appropriate person/authority any conscientious objection relative to professional practice	–	–	100	–	–
3. Ensure the adequacy of resources	–	–	50	50	–
4. Make known to an appropriate person/authority circumstances which militate against safe standards of practice	–	–	50	50	–
5. Have regard to the workload on colleagues	–	–	50	50	–

	Completely	To a reasonable degree	On the whole Yes	Not usually	Impossible
6. Have regard to the workload on subordinates	–	–	50	50	–
7. Have regard to the pressures on colleagues	–	–	50	50	–
8. Have regard to the pressures on subordinates	–	–	50	50	–
9. Take action to reduce the workload on colleagues	–	–	50	50	–
10. Take action to reduce the workload on subordinates	–	–	50	50	–
11. Take action to reduce undue pressures on colleagues	–	–	50	50	–
12. Take action to reduce the pressures on subordinates	–	–	50	50	–

Educational

	Completely	To a reasonable degree	On the whole Yes	Not usually	Impossible
1. Improve own professional competence – skills and knowledge (specific)	–	–	–	100	–
2. Assist colleagues to develop professional competence (skills and knowledge)	–	–	50	50	–

	Completely	To a reasonable degree	On the whole Yes	Not usually	Impossible
3. Assist subordinates to develop professional competence (passing on of skills and knowledge)	–	50	50	–	–
4. Teach subordinates	–	–	100	–	–
5. Advise patients (health education)	–	–	–	50	50
6. Counsel staff as appropriate	–	–	–	50	50
7. Ensure own professional development (general)	–	–	–	100	–
8. Prepare programmes of training (nursing techniques and ward management)	–	–	100	–	–
9. Act as assessor (ward-based examinations)	–	–	–	–	–

PROFESSIONAL BODY

Clinical ($n=1$)

Q. The following is a list of responsibilities defined by the UKCC and Senior Nurse Management in relation to the job of the professional nurse. Indicate how far it is possible to meet these responsibilities in doing their job ($\sqrt{}$ = response)

	Completely	To a reasonable degree	On the whole Yes	Not usually	Impossible
1. Act always to promote and safeguard the wellbeing of patients			$\sqrt{}$		
2. Take account of the customs of patients			$\sqrt{}$		

	Completely	To a reasonable degree	On the whole Yes	Not usually	Impossible
3. Carry out medical instructions		√			
4. Ensure high standards of care				√	
5. Respect the confidential information of patients			√		
6. Ensure safe standards of practice (supervision of work)				√	
7. Inform persons as appropriate of patient's progress (relatives, doctor, senior nursing manager)			√		

Managerial

	Completely	To a reasonable degree	On the whole Yes	Not usually	Impossible
1. Work in a collaborative manner with other health-care professionals			√		
2. Make known to an appropriate person/authority any conscientious objection relative to professional practice				√	
3. Ensure the adequacy of resources					√
4. Make known to an appropriate person/authority circumstances which militate against safe standards of practice					√

	Completely	To a reasonable degree	On the whole Yes	Not usually	Impossible
5. Have regard to the workload on colleagues				√	
6. Have regard to the workload on subordinates				√	
7. Have regard to the pressures on colleagues				√	
8. Have regard to the pressures on subordinates				√	
9. Take action to reduce the workload on colleagues					√
10. Take action to reduce the workload on subordinates					√
11. Take action to reduce undue pressures on colleagues				√	
12. Take action to reduce the pressures on subordinates					√

Educational

	Completely	To a reasonable degree	On the whole Yes	Not usually	Impossible
1. Improve own professional competence – skills and knowledge (specific)			√		
2. Assist colleagues to develop professional competence (skills and knowledge)		√			

	Completely	To a reasonable degree	On the whole Yes	Not usually	Impossible
3. Assist subordinates to develop professional competence (passing on of skills and knowledge)			√		
4. Teach subordinates			√		
5. Advise patients (health education)				√	
6. Counsel staff as appropriate				√	
7. Ensure own professional development (general)				√	
8. Prepare programmes of training (nursing techniques and ward management)			√		
9. Act as assessor (ward-based examinations)	–	–	–	–	–

APPENDIX E

RATING BY NURSES AND OTHER PROFESSIONALS OF THE EXTENT TO WHICH PATIENTS' NEEDS WERE MET

WARD SISTER $(n=21)$

Q. From the following general list of patient needs indicate to what extent you are able to meet these needs during a patient's stay in hospital.

	Great extent	Fair extent	Some extent	Inadequately
1. Belongingness (helping the patient adjust to the ward group)	28.57	47.62	4.76	19.05
2. Comfort (general)	52.38	42.86	–	4.76
3. Confidentiality	95.24	4.76	–	–
4. Dignity (self-respect)	61.90	23.81	9.52	4.76
5. Emotional (reassurance – reduction of fear and anxiety	47.62	47.62	–	4.76
6. Friendliness (ward staff)	80.95	14.29	–	4.76
7. Identity (recognition of patient as a person – individual)	76.19	14.29	4.76	4.76
8. Information (care, progress, ward procedure)	57.14	28.57	9.52	4.76
9. Independence	57.14	23.81	4.76	14.29
10. Likes and dislikes (within reason)	33.33	52.38	9.52	4.76
11. Pain relief	90.48	9.32	–	–

	Great extent	Fair extent	Some extent	Inadequately
12. Personal hygiene	76.19	23.81	–	–
13. Physical (food, drink, bodily protection)	61.90	33.33	–	4.76
14. Privacy	23.81	57.14	4.76	14.29
15. Rest	33.33	57.14	4.76	4.76
16. Safety	61.90	28.57	4.76	4.76
17. Sleep	23.81	61.9	4.76	9.52
18. Religious practice (ensuring a visit by the hospital chaplain; attending religious service)	85.71	4.76	–	9.52
19. Talking to patient (informally)	38.1	38.1	19.05	4.76

STAFF NURSE ($n = 74$)

Q. From the following general list of patient needs indicate to what extent you are able to meet these needs during a patient's stay in hospital.

	Great extent	Fair extent	Some extent	Inadequately
1. Belongingness (helping the patient adjust to the ward group)	89.19	9.46	1.35	–
2. Comfort (general)	56.76	39.19	4.05	–
3. Confidentiality	36.49	62.16	1.35	–
4. Dignity (self-respect)	94.59	5.41	–	–
5. Emotional (reassurance – reduction of fear and anxiety)	68.92	27.03	2.7	1.35
6. Friendliness (ward staff)	58.11	33.78	4.05	4.05
7. Identity (recognition of patient as a person – individual)	40.54	54.05	2.70	2.70

	Great extent	Fair extent	Some extent	Inadequately
8. Information (care, progress, ward procedure)	31.08	66.22	2.70	–
9. Independence	85.14	13.51	1.35	–
10. Likes and dislikes (within reason)	93.24	6.76	–	–
11. Pain relief	56.76	36.49	5.41	1.35
12. Personal hygiene	21.63	54.05	20.27	4.05
13. Physical (food, drink, bodily protection)	13.51	64.86	20.27	1.35
14. Privacy	59.46	37.84	2.7	–
15. Rest	8.22	69.86	20.55	1.37
16. Safety	75.68	16.22	2.7	–
17. Sleep	34.49	44.59	10.81	8.11
18. Religious practice (ensuring a visit by the hospital chaplain; attending religious service)	39.19	60.81	–	–
19. Talking to patient (informally)	24.32	75.68	–	–

UNIT NURSE MANAGER ($n = 6$)

Q. From the following list of patients' needs indicate to what extent nurses are able to meet these needs during a patient's stay in hospital.

	Great extent	Fair extent	Some extent	Inadequately
1. Belongingness (helping the patient adjust to the ward group)	–	83.33	16.66	–
2. Comfort (general)	66.66	33.33	–	–
3. Confidentiality	100	–	–	–

	Great extent	Fair extent	Some extent	Inadequately
4. Dignity (self-respect)	83.33	–	16.66	–
5. Emotional (reassurance – reduction of fear and anxiety)	33.33	66.66	–	–
6. Friendliness (ward staff)	100	–	–	–
7. Identity (recognition of patient as a person – individual)	33.33	66.66	–	–
8. Information (care, progress, ward procedure)	50	50	–	–
9. Independence	50	33.33	16.66	–
10. Likes and dislikes (within reason)	16.66	66.66	16.66	–
11. Pain relief	66.66	33.33	–	–
12. Personal hygiene	83.33	16.66	–	–
13. Physical (food, drink, bodily protection)	83.33	16.66	–	–
14. Privacy	33.33	50	16.66	–
15. Rest	16.66	66.66	16.66	
16. Safety	50	50	–	–
17. Sleep	33.33	50	16.66	–
18. Religious practice (ensuring a visit by the hospital chaplain; attending religious service)	100	–	–	–
19. Talking to patient (informally)	50	50	–	–

SENIOR NURSE MANAGER ($n = 2$)

Q. From the following list of patients' needs indicate to what extent nurses are able to meet these needs during a patient's stay in hospital.

	Great extent	Fair extent	Some extent	Inadequately
1. Belongingness (helping the patient adjust to the ward group)	50	50	–	–
2. Comfort (general)	50	50	–	–
3. Confidentiality	100	–	–	–
4. Dignity (self-respect)	50	50	–	–
5. Emotional (reassurance – reduction of fear and anxiety)	50	50	–	–
6. Friendliness (ward staff)	50	50	–	–
7. Identity (recognition of patient as a person – individual)	100	–	–	–
8. Information (care, progress, ward procedure)	–	100	–	–
9. Independence	–	100	–	–
10. Likes and dislikes (within reason)	–	50	50	–
11. Pain relief	–	100	–	–
12. Personal hygiene	50	50	–	–
13. Physical (food, drink, bodily protection)	50	50	–	–
14. Privacy	–	100	–	–
15. Rest	–	50	50	–
16. Safety	–	100	–	–
17. Sleep	–	–	100	–

	Great extent	Fair extent	Some extent	Inadequately
18. Religious practice (ensuring a visit by the hospital chaplain; attending religious service)	–	50	50	–
19. Talking to patient (informally)	–	50	50	–

DOCTOR $(n=29)$

Q. From the following list of patients' needs indicate to what extent nurses are able to meet these needs during a patient's stay in hospital.

	Great extent	Fair extent	Some extent	Inadequately
1. Belongingness (helping the patient adjust to the ward group)	24.13	27.58	41.37	6.89
2. Comfort (general)	17.24	68.96	13.79	–
3. Confidentiality	24.13	55.17	17.24	3.44
4. Dignity (self-respect)	17.24	51.72	20.68	10.34
5. Emotional (reassurance – reduction of fear and anxiety)	34.48	44.82	20.64	–
6. Friendliness (ward staff)	72.41	24.13	3.44	–
7. Identity (recognition of patient as a person – individual)	37.93	44.82	13.79	3.44
8. Information (care, progress, ward procedure)	17.24	48.27	27.58	6.89
9. Independence	13.79	55.17	24.13	6.89
10. Likes and dislikes (within reason)	6.89	62.06	17.24	13.79
11. Pain relief	65.31	20.68	10.34	3.44
12. Personal hygiene	62.06	34.48	–	3.44

	Great extent	Fair extent	Some extent	Inadequately
13. Physical (food, drink, bodily protection)	27.58	62.06	10.34	–
14. Privacy	3.44	34.48	37.93	24.13
15. Rest	10.34	41.37	37.93	10.34
16. Safety	24.13	65.51	10.34	–
17. Sleep	3.44	44.82	37.93	13.79
18. Religious practice (ensuring a visit by the hospital chaplain; attending religious service)	34.48	27.58	20.68	10.34
19. Talking to patient (informally)	20.68	17.24	37.93	24.13

OFFICERS OF THE UKCC OR ENB $n=2$)

Q. From the following list of patients' needs indicate to what extent nurses are able to meet these needs during a patient's stay in hospital.

	Great extent	Fair extent	Some extent	Inadequately
1. Belonging (helping the patient adjust to the ward group)	–	–	100	–
2. Comfort (general)	–	100	–	–
3. Confidentiality	–	50	50	–
4. Dignity (self-respect)	–	–	50	50
5. Emotional (reassurance – reduction of fear and anxiety)	–	100	–	–
6. Friendliness (ward staff)	100	–	–	–
7. Identity (recognition of patient as a person – individual)	–	50	50	–
8. Information (care, progress, ward procedure)	–	–	100	–

	Great extent	Fair extent	Some extent	Inadequately
9. Independence	–	–	100	–
10. Likes and dislikes (within reason)	–	–	100	–
11. Pain relief	50	50	–	–
12. Personal hygiene	100	–	–	–
13. Physical (food, drink, bodily protection)	–	100	–	–
14. Privacy	–	–	100	–
15. Rest	–	–	100	–
16. Safety	–	–	100	–
17. Sleep	–	–	100	–
18. Religious practice (ensuring a visit by the hospital chaplain; attending religious service)	–	–	–	–
19. Talking to patient (informally)	–	50	–	50

OFFICER OF THE RCN ($n=1$)

Q. From the following list of patients' needs indicate to what extent nurses are able to meet these needs during a patient's stay in hospital. ($\sqrt{}$ = response)

	Great extent	Fair extent	Some extent	Inadequately
1. Belongingness (helping the patient adjust to the ward group)		$\sqrt{}$		
2. Comfort (general)		$\sqrt{}$		
3. Confidentiality				$\sqrt{}$
4. Dignity (self-respect)				$\sqrt{}$

	Great extent	Fair extent	Some extent	Inadequately
5. Emotional (reassurance – reduction of fear and anxiety)			√	
6. Friendliness (ward staff)		√		
7. Identity (recognition of patient as a person – individual)			√	
8. Information (care, progress, ward procedure)				√
9. Independence			√	
10. Likes and dislikes (within reason)		√		
11. Pain relief		√		
12. Personal hygiene	√			
13. Physical (food, drink, bodily protection)		√		
14. Privacy				√
15. Rest				√
16. Safety				√
17. Sleep				√
18. Religious practice (ensuring a visit by the hospital chaplain; attending religious service)				–
19. Talking to patient (informally)				√

References

Preface

Audit Commission (1991) *the Virtue of Patients: Making Best Use of Ward Nursing Resources* (Audit Commission, National Health Service Report No. 4), HMSO, London.

Audit Commission (1992) *Making Time for Patients: A Handbook for Ward Sisters* (Audit Commission, National Health Service Handbook), HMSO, London.

Bowman, M.P. (1990) An exploration of the role of the nurse in acute medical and surgical and longstay (geriatric) wards. University of Newcastle upon Tyne, Newcastle upon Tyne, PhD thesis.

Department of Health (1989a) *Caring for People: Community Care in the Next Decade and Beyond* (Cm. 849), HMSO, London.

Department of Health (1989b) *Self-governing Hospitals: an Initial Guide* (Cm. 555), HMSO, London.

English National Board for Nursing Midwifery and Health Visiting (1992) *ENB News*, **Spring/Summer/Autumn**, ENB, London.

European Economic Community (1977) Nursing Directives, 77/452/EEC, 77/453/EEC, 77/454/EEC. *Official Journal of the European Communities*, **20**, 1–11.

European Economic Community (1989) Nursing directives, 89/594/EEC, 89/595/EEC. *Official Journal of the European Communities*, **32**, 19–29.

Fowler, N. (Secretary of State for Health) (1983) *Nurses, Midwives and Health Visitors, Rules Approval Order* (No. 873), HMSO, London.

Hingley, P. *et al.* (1984) *Stress (Report of the King Edward Hospitals Fund)* (Project Paper No. 60), King Edward Hospitals Fund, London.

Hingley, P. and Cooper, C.G. (1986) *Stress and the Nurse Manager*, John Wiley & Sons Ltd., Chichester.

Marshall, J. (1980) Stress amongst nurses, in *White Collar and Professional Stress*, John Wiley & Sons Ltd., Chichester.

National Health Service and Community Care Act 1990 (Chapter 19), HMSO, London.

Nurses, Midwives and Health Visitors Act 1979 (Chapter 36), HMSO, London.

Revans, R.W. (1964) *Standards for Morale: Cause and Effect in Hospitals*, Oxford University Press, Oxford.

Royal College of Nursing of the United Kingdom (1984) *A Report of the Effects of the Financial and Manpower Cuts in the NHS (Nurse Alert)*, RCN, London.

Seccombe, I. and Ball, J. (1992) *Motivation, Morale and Mobility: A Profile of Qualified Nurses in the 1990s.* (IMS Report No. 233), RCN, London.

United Kingdom, Central Council for Nursing, Midwifery and Health Visiting (1984) *Code of Professional Conduct for Nurses, Midwives and Health Visitors*, 2nd edn, UKCC, London.

United Kingdom Central Council for Nursing, Midwifery and Health Visiting (1986) *Project 2000 (Report)*, UKCC, London.

United Kingdom Central Council for Nursing, Midwifery and Health Visiting (1987) *Project 2000: How Does It Affect Your Future?* UKCC, London.

United Kingdom Central Council for Nursing, Midwifery and Health Visiting (1992) *The Scope of Professional Practice*, UKCC, London.

Chapter 1

Benne, K.D. and Bennis, W. (1959) Role confusion and conflict in nursing. *American Journal of Nursing*, **LIX**(2), 196–8; **LIX**(3), 380–3.

Bowman, M.P. (1990) An exploration of the role of the nurse in acute medical and surgical and longstay (geriatric) wards, University of Newcastle upon Tyne, Newcastle upon Tyne, England, PhD Thesis.

Briggs, A. (Chairman) (1972) *Report of the Committee on Nursing* (Cm. 5115), HMSO, London.

Department of Health and Social Security (1972) *Management Arrangements for the Reorganised National Health Service* (grey book), HMSO, London.

Department of Health and Social Security (1979) *Patients First.* Consultative paper on structure and management of the National Health Service in England and Wales, HMSO, London.

Department of Health Nursing Division (1989) *A Strategy for Nursing* (a report of the Steering Committee), Department of Health Nursing Division, London.

Department of Health and Social Security (1991) *The Patient's Charter*, HMSO, London.

European Economic Community (1977) Nursing Directives, 77/452/EEC, 77/453/EEC, 77/454/EEC. *Official Journal of the European Communities*, **20**, 1–12.

European Economic Community (1989) Nursing directives, 89/594/EEC, 89/595/EEC. *Official Journal of the European Communities*, **32**, 19–29.

Griffiths, R. (Chairman) (1983) *National Health Service Management Inquiry*, DHSS, London.

Health Services Act 1980 (Chapter 53), HMSO, London.

Horder, T.J. (First Baron Horder of Ashford; Chairman) (1943) *Report of the Nursing Reconstruction Committee*, Royal College of Nursing of the United Kingdom, London.

International Council of Nurses (1965) Special and Committee Reports presented to the ICN Board of Directors and Grand Council Meetings, Frankfurt.

Judge, H. (Chairman) (1985) *The Education of Nurses: a New Dispensation* (Commission on Nursing Education), RCN, London.

Leonard, A. and Jowett, S. (1990) Charting the course: A study of the 6 ENB pilot schemes in pre-registration nurse education (Research paper No. 1), National Foundation for Educational Research, Berks.

McFarlane, Professor Baroness (1983) Mirror mirror on the wall (Nursing Mirror lecture, 1983). *Nursing Mirror*, **156**(23), 17–20.

Merrison, A. (Chairman) (1979) *Royal Commission on the National Health Service* (Cm. 7615), HMSO, London.

Platt, H. (Chairman) (1964) *A Reform of Nursing Education*, Royal College of Nursing of the United Kingdom, London.

Nurses, Midwives and Health Visitors Act 1979 (Chapter 36), HMSO, London.

Nurses, Midwives and Health Visitors Rules Approval Order 1983 (No. 873), HMSO, London.

Powell, M. (Chairman) (1966) *The Post Certificate Training and Education of Nurses*, HMSO, London.

Price Waterhouse (1987) *Project 2000: Report on the Costs, Benefits and Manpower Implications*, UKCC, London.

Revans, R.W. (1964) *Standards for Morale: Cause and Effect in Hospitals*, Oxford University Press, Oxford.

Royal College of Nursing of the United Kingdom (1981) *Towards Standards* (Discussion document), RCN, London.

Royal College of Nursing of the United Kingdom (1982) Advanced clinical roles (Seminar), RCN, London.

Royal College of Nursing of the United Kingdom (1983) *Towards a New Professional Structure for Nursing*, RCN, London.

Royal College of Nursing of the United Kingdom (1988) *Boundaries of Nursing: a Policy Statement*, RCN, London.

Salmon, B. (Chairman) (1966) *Report of the committee on senior nursing staff structure*, HMSO, London.

Tolliday, H. (1972) Defining the nurse's role (occasional paper). *Nursing Times*, **68**(14), 53–6.

United Kingdom Central Council for Nursing, Midwifery and Health Visiting (1986) *Project 2000* (Report), UKCC, London.

United Kingdom Central Council for Nursing, Midwifery and Health Visiting (1992a) *Code of Professional Conduct*, UKCC, London.

United Kingdom Central Council for Nursing, Midwifery and Health Visiting (1992b) *The Scope of Professional Practice*, UKCC, London.

Chapter 2

Anderson, E.R. (1973) *The Role of the Nurse*, Royal College of Nursing Research Project, Series 2, No. 1, RCN, London.

Banton, M. (1968) *Roles: an Introduction to the Study of Social Relations*, Tavistock Publications, London.

Batey, M.V. and Lewis, F.M. (1982) Clarifying autonomy and accountability. *Journal of Nursing Administration*, **XII**(9), 13–18; **XII**(10), 10–15.

Brown, W. (1971) *Exploration in Management*, Penguin Books, London.

Cang, S. *et al.* (1981) *An Emerging Model for Ward Sister Roles in General Hospitals* (North West Thames Regional Nursing Project), Health Services Organisation Research Unit, Brunel University, London.

Goldstone, L.A. (1983) *'Monitor': an Index of Quality of Nursing Care for Acute*

Medical and Surgical Wards, Newcastle upon Tyne Polytechnic Products Ltd., Newcastle upon Tyne.

Hardy, M.E. and Conway, M.E. (1978) *Role Theory: Perspectives for Health Professionals*, Appleton-Century Crofts, New York.

Junker, B.H. (1960) *Fieldwork: an Introduction to the Social Sciences*, University of Chicago Press, Chicago.

Kraegel, J.M. *et al.* (1972) A system of care based on patient needs. *Nursing Outlook*, **20**(4), 257–64.

Kramer, M.F. (1966) Some effects of exposure to employing bureaucracies on the role conceptions and role deprivation of neophyte collegiate nurses. Stanford University. Dissertation.

Kramer, M.F. (1974) *Reality Shock: Why Nurses Leave Nursing*, C.V. Mosby Co., Saint Louis.

McDougall, W. (1969) *An Outline of Psychology*, Methuen and Co. Ltd., London.

Merton, R.K. (1967) *On Theoretical Sociology*, The Free Press, New York.

Mintzberg, H. (1968) The manager at work – determining the activities, roles, and programs by structured observation, MIT Sloan School of Management, Cambridge, MA. PhD Thesis.

Mintzberg, H. (1970) Structured observation as a method to study managerial work. *Journal of Management Studies*, **7**, 87–104.

Mintzberg, H. (1971) Managerial work: analysis from observation. *Management Science*, **18**(2), 97–110.

Mintzberg, H. (1973) *The Nature of Managerial Work*, Harper & Row, New York.

Nord, W.R. (ed.) (1972) *Concepts and Controversy by Organizational Behavior*, Goodyear Publishing Company, Inc., CA.

Patton, M.Q. (1978) *Qualitative Evaluation Methods*, Sage Publications, London.

Pembrey, S. (1980) *The Ward Sister – Key to Nursing* (Royal College of Nursing research report), RCN, London.

Salmon, B. (Chairman) (1966) *Committee on Senior Nursing Staff Structure*, HMSO, London.

United Kingdom Central Council for Nursing, Midwifery and Health Visiting (1984) *Code of Professional Conduct for Nurses, Midwives and Health Visitors*, UKCC, London.

United Kingdom Central Council for Nursing, Midwifery and Health Visiting (1986) *Project 2000 Report*, UKCC, London.

Whitmore, D.A. (1971) *Measurement and Control of Work*, Heinemann, London.

Whitmore, D.A. (1973) *Work Study and Related Management Services*, 3rd edn, Heinemann, London.

Williams, D. (1969) The administrative contribution of the nursing sister. *Journal of Public Administration*, **XLVIII**, 307–28.

Chapter 3

Aiken, L.H. (1981) Nursing priorities for the 1980s: hospitals and nursing homes. *American Journal of Nursing*, **81**(2), 324–30.

Anderson, E.R. (1973) *The Role of the Nurse* (RCN nursing research project), series 2, No. 1. RCN, London.

Audit Commission (1991) *The Virtue of Patients: Making Best Use of Ward Nursing Resources* (Audit Commission National Health Service Report No. 4), HMSO, London.

Audit Commission (1992) *Making Time for Patients: A Handbook for Ward Sisters* (Audit Commission National Health Service Handbook), HMSO, London.

Briggs, A.D. (Chairman) (1972) *Report of the Committee on Nursing* (Cm. 5115), HMSO, London.

Cang, S. *et al.* (1981) *An Emerging Model for Ward Sister Roles in General Hospitals* (North West Thames Regional Nursing Project), Health Services Organisation Research Unit, Brunel University, Middlesex.

Department of Health (1989) *Working for Patients* (White Paper, Cm. 555), HMSO, London.

Department of Health and Social Security (1979) *Patients First* (Consultative paper on the structure and management of the National Health Service in England and Wales), HMSO, London.

Department of Health Nursing Division (1989) *A Strategy for Nursing* (a report of the Steering Committee), Department of Health, London.

Earl of Crawford and Balcarres (Chairman) (1932) *The Lancet Commission on Nursing* (Final report), The Lancet Ltd., London.

Goldstone, L.A. (1983) '*Monitor*': *An Index of Quality of Nursing Care for Acute Medical and Surgical Wards*, Newcastle upon Tyne Polytechnic Products Ltd., Newcastle upon Tyne.

Hardy, M.E. and Conway, M.E. (1978) *Role Theory: Perspectives for Health Professionals*, Appleton-Century Croft, New York.

Hingley, P. *et al.* (1984) *Stress* (*A Report of the King Edward Hospitals Fund*) (Project Paper No. 60), King Edward Hospitals Fund, London.

Hingley, P. and Cooper, C.G. (1986) *Stress and the Nurse Manager*, Wiley & Sons Ltd., Chichester.

Judge, H. (Chairman) (1985) *The Education of Nurses: A Dispensation* (Commission on Nursing Education), RCN, London.

Kraegel, J.M. *et al.* (1972) A system of care based on patient needs. *Nursing Outlook*, **20**(4), 257–64.

Kramer, M.F. (1966) Some effects of exposure to employing bureaucracies on the role conceptions and role deprivation of neophyte collegiate nurses, Stanford University, PhD thesis.

Kramer, M.F. (1974) *Reality Shock: Why Nurses Leave Nursing*, C.V. Mosby Co., St Louis.

Marshall, J. (1980) Stress amongst nurses, in *White Collar and Professional stress* (eds C.L. Cooper and J. Marshall), Wiley, Chichester.

Mayeroff, M. (1971) *On Caring*, Harper and Row, New York.

Mayston, E.L. (Chairman) (1969) *Report of the Working Party on Structure in the Local Authority Nursing Service*, DHSS, London.

Merrison, A. (Chairman) (1979) *Royal Commission on the National Health Service* (Cm. 7615), HMSO, London.

Nursing and Midwifery Staff Negotiating Council (1988) *A Guide to the Clinical Grading Structure*, Nursing and Midwifery Staff Negotiating Council, London.

Price Waterhouse (1987) *Project 2000: Report on the Costs, Benefits, and Manpower Implications of Project 2000*, UKCC, London.

Revans, R. (1964) *Standards of Morale: Cause and Effect in Hospitals*, Oxford University Press, Oxford.

Rowbottom, R. and Billis, D. (1987) *Organisational Design*, Gower Publishing Co. Ltd, England.

Royal College of Nursing of the United Kingdom (1981) *Towards Standards* (*Discussion Document*) (Second Report of the RCN Working Party on Standards of Nursing Care (England & Wales), RCN, London.

Royal College of Nursing of the United Kingdom (1984) *Nurse Alert: A Report of the Effects of the Financial and Manpower Cuts in the NHS*, RCN, London.

Royal College of Nursing of the United Kingdom (1988) *Boundaries of Nursing: A Policy Statement*, RCN, London.

Salmon, B. (Chairman) (1966) *Committee on Senior Nursing Structure*, HMSO, London.

Taylor, C.D. (1962) Sociological sheep shearing. *Nursing Forum*, **1**, 79–100.

United Kingdom Central Council for Nursing, Midwifery and Health Visiting (1984) *Code of Professional Conduct for Nurses, Midwives and Health Visitors*, 2nd edn, UKCC, London.

United Kingdom Central Council for Nursing, Midwifery and Health Visiting (1986) *Project 2000 (A Review of the Professional Preparation for Nursing, Midwifery and Health Visiting)*, UKCC, London.

United Kingdom Central Council for Nursing, Midwifery and Health Visiting (1989) *Exercising Accountability: A Framework to Assist Nurses, Midwives and Health Visitors to Consider the Ethical Aspects of Professional Practice*, UKCC, London.

United Kingdom Central Council for Nursing, Midwifery and Health Visiting (1992a) *The Code of Professional Conduct*, UKCC, London.

United Kingdom Central Council for Nursing, Midwifery and Health Visiting (1992b) *The Scope of Professional Practice*, UKCC, London.

Visser, A.P. (1984) *Experience of Patients During their Stay in a General Hospital*, Van Gorcum, Assen, pp. 280–2.

Wieland, G.F. (ed.) (1981) *Improving Health Care Management: Organization Development and Organization Change*, Health Administration Press, Ann Arbor, MI.

World Health Organization (1966) *WHO Expert Committee on Nursing. Fifth report* (WHO Technical Report Series No. 347), WHO, Geneva.

Chapter 4

Aiken, L.H. (1981) Nursing priorities for the 1980's: hospitals and nursing homes. *American Journal of Nursing*, **81**(2), 324–30.

Briggs, A. (Chairman) (1972) *Report of the Committee on Nursing* (Cm. 5115), HMSO, London.

Department of Health (1989) *Self Governing Hospitals: An Initial Guide*, HMSO, London.

Hingley, P. *et al.* (1984) *Stress* (Report of the King Edward Hospitals Fund), Project Paper No. 60, King Edward Hospitals Fund, London.

Hingley, P. and Cooper, C.G. (1986) *Stress and the Nurse Manager*, Wiley & Sons, Chichester.

Katz, D. and Kahn, R.L. (1966) *The Social Psychology of Organizations*, 2nd edn, Wiley, New York.

Martinko, M.J. and Gardner, W.L. (1985) Beyond structured observations: methodological issues and new directions. *Academic Management Review*, **10**(4), 676–95.

Mayston, E.L. (Chairman) (1969) *Report of the Working Party on Structure in the Local Authority Nursing Service*, DHSS, London.

Merrison, A. (Chairman) (1979) *Royal Commission on the National Health Service* (Cm. 7615), HMSO, London.

National Health Service and Community Care Act 1990, HMSO, London.

Pembrey, S. (1980) The ward sister – key to nursing (Royal College of Nursing research report), RCN, London.

Royal College of Nursing of the United Kingdom (1984) *Nurse Alert: A Report of the Effects of the Financial and Manpower Cuts in the NHS*, RCN, London.

Royal College of Nursing of the United Kingdom (1988) *Boundaries of Nursing: A Policy Statement*, RCN, London.

Salmon, B. (Chairman) (1966) *Committee on Senior Nursing Staff Structure*, HMSO, London.

Seccombe, I. and Ball, J. (1992) *Motivation, Morale and Mobility: A Profile of Qualified Nurses in the 1990's* (IMS Report No. 233), RCN, London.

United Kingdom Central Council for Nursing, Midwifery and Health Visiting (1985) *Introducing Project 2000* (Project Paper 1), UKCC, London.

United Kingdom Central Council for Nursing, Midwifery and Health Visiting (1989) *Exercising Accountability: A Framework to Assist Nurses, Midwives and Health Visitors to Consider Ethical Aspects of Professional Practice*, UKCC, London.

United Kingdom Central Council for Nursing, Midwifery and Health Visiting (1992) *The Scope of Professional Practice*, UKCC, London.

Chapter 5

Audit Commission (1991) *The Virtue of Patients: Making Best Use of Ward Nursing Resources*, HMSO, London.

Audit Commission (1992) *Making Time for Patients: A Handbook for Ward Sisters*, HMSO, London.

Batey, M.V. and Lewis, F.M. (1982) Clarifying autonomy and accountability in nursing service (Parts 1 and 2). *Journal of Nursing Administration*, **XII**(9), 13–18; (10), 10–15.

Briggs, A.D. (Chairman) (1972) *Report of the Committee on Nursing* (Cm. 5115), HMSO, London.

Davidmann, D. (1984) *Reorganising the National Health Service: An Evaluation of the Griffiths Report*, Social Organisation Ltd, Middlesex.

Department of Health Nursing Division (1989) *A Strategy for Nursing* (A report of the Steering Committee), DoH Nursing Division, London.

Department of Health and Social Security (1984) *Implementation of the NHS Management Inquiry* (*HC(84)13*, HMSO, London.

European Economic Community (1977) Nursing Directives 77/452/EEC, 77/453/EEC, 77/454/EEC. *Official Journal of the European Community*, **20**, 1–11.

European Economic Community (1989) Nursing Directives, 89/594/EEC, 89/595/EEC. *Official Journal of the European Community*, **32**, 19–29.

Evans, T. and Maxwell, R. (1984) *Griffiths: Challenge and Response* (*Evidence to the Select Committee on Social Services, 1984*), King Edward's Hospital Fund for London, London.

Griffiths, R. (Chairman) (1983) *NHS Management Inquiry*, DHSS, London.

Hall, R.A. (1968) Professionalization and bureaucratization. *American Social Review*, **93**, 92–104.

Hardy, M.E. and Conway, M.E. (1978) *Role Theory: Perspectives for Health Professionals*, Appleton–Century Croft, New York.

Lanara, V.A. (1982) Responsibility in nursing. *International Nursing Review*, **29**(1), 7–10.

Mayeroff, M. (1971) *On Caring*, Harper & Row, New York.

Merrison, A. (Chairman) (1979) *Royal Commission on the National Health Service* (Cm. 7615), HMSO, London.

Nurses, Midwives and Health Visitors Act 1979 (Chapter 36), HMSO, London.

Pyne, R. (1985) Trends in accountability. *Senior Nurse*, **2**(1), 14–15.

Rowbottom, R. and Billis, D. (1987) *Organisational Design*, Gower, London.

Royal College of Nursing of the United Kingdom (1982) Advanced clinical roles (seminar), RCN, London.

Royal College of Nursing of the United Kingdom (1983) *Towards a Professional Structure for Nursing* (Report of the Working Group on a professional nursing structure for the NHS), RCN, London.

Royal College of Nursing of the United Kingdom (1988) *Boundaries of Nursing: A Policy Statement*, RCN, London.

Salmon, B. (Chairman) (1966) *Committee on Senior Nursing Staff Structure*, HMSO, London.

Seccombe, I. and Ball, J. (1992) *Motivation, Morale and Mobility: A Profile of Qualified Nurses in the 1990's* (IMS Report No. 233), RCN, London.

United Kingdom Central Council for Nursing, Midwifery and Health Visiting (1984) *Code of Professional Conduct for Nurses, Midwives and Health Visitors*, 2nd edn, UKCC, London.

United Kingdom Central Council for Nursing, Midwifery and Health Visiting (1987) *Confidentiality: An Elaboration of Clause 9 of the Second Edition of the UKCC's Code of Professional Conduct for the Nurse, Midwife and Health Visitor* (Advisory document), UKCC, London.

United Kingdom Central Council for Nursing, Midwifery and Health Visiting (1989) *Exercising Accountability: A Framework to Assist Nurses, Midwives and Health Visitors to Consider Ethical Aspects of Professional Practice* (advisory document), UKCC, London.

United Kingdom Central Council for Nursing, Midwifery and Health Visiting (1992) *Code of Professional Conduct for Nurses, Midwives and Health Visitors*, UKCC, London.

United Kingdom Central Council for Nursing, Midwifery and Health Visiting (1992) *The Scope of Professional Practice*, UKCC, London.

Chapter 6

Audit Commission (1991) *The Virtue of Patients: Making Best Use of Ward Nursing Resources*, HMSO, London.

REFERENCES

Audit Commission (1992) *Making Time for Patients: A Handbook for Ward Sisters*, HMSO, London.

Batey, M.V. and Lewis, F.M. (1982) Clarifying autonomy and accountability in nursing service (parts 1 and 2). *Journal of Nursing Administration*, **XII**(9), 13–18; (10) 10–15.

Briggs, A.D. (Chairman) (1972) *Report of the Committee on Nursing* (Cm. 5115), HMSO, London.

Department of Health Nursing Division (1989) *A Strategy for Nursing* (A report of the Steering Committee), DoH Nursing Division, London.

Engel, G.V. (1970) Professional autonomy and bureaucratic organization. *Administrative Science Quarterly*, **15**, 12–21.

European Economic Community (1977) Nursing Directives 77/452/EEC, 77/453/EEC, 77/454/EEC. *Official Journal of the European Community*, **20**, 1–11.

European Economic Community (1989) Nursing Directives, 89/594/EEC, 89/595/EEC. *Official Journal of the European Community*, **32**, 19–29.

Hall, R.H. (1968) Professionalization and bureaucratization. *American Sociological Review*, **33**(1), 92–104.

Mayeroff, M. (1971) *On Caring*, Harper & Row, New York.

Merrison, A. (Chairman) (1979) *Royal Commission on the National Health Service* (Cm. 7615), HMSO, London.

Nurses, Midwives and Health Visitors Act 1979 (Chapter 36), HMSO, London.

Rowbottom, R. and Billis, D. (1987) *Organisation Design*, Gower Publishing, Aldershot.

Royal College of Nursing of the United Kingdom (1982) *Advanced Clinical Roles* (seminar), RCN, London.

Royal College of Nursing of the United Kingdom (1983) *Towards a Professional Structure for Nursing* (Report of a working group on a professional nursing structure for the NHS), RCN, London.

Royal College of Nursing of the United Kingdom (1988) *Boundaries of Nursing: A Policy Statement*, RCN, London.

Salmon, B. (Chairman) (1966) *Committee on Senior Nursing Staff Structure*, HMSO, London.

United Kingdom Central Council for Nursing, Midwifery and Health Visiting (1986) *Project 2000: A New Preparation for Practice*, UKCC, London.

United Kingdom Central Council for Nursing, Midwifery and Health Visiting (1987) *Confidentiality: An Elaboration of Clause 9 of the Second Edition of the UKCC's Code of Professional Conduct for the Nurse, Midwife and Health Visitor* (advisory paper), UKCC, London.

United Kingdom Central Council for Nursing, Midwifery and Health Visiting (1989) *Exercising Accountability: A Framework to Assist Nurses, Midwives and Health Visitors to Consider Ethical Aspects of Professional Practice* (advisory document), UKCC, London.

United Kingdom Central Council for Nursing, Midwifery and Health Visiting (1992a) *Code of Professional Conduct for the Nurse, Midwife and Health Visitor*, UKCC, London.

United Kingdom Central Council for Nursing, Midwifery and Health Visiting (1992b) *The Scope of Professional Practice*, UKCC, London.

Chapter 7

Audit Commission (1991) *The Virtue of Patients: Making Best Use of Ward Nursing Resources* (Audit Commission National Health Service Report No. 4), HMSO, London.

Audit Commission (1992) *Making Time for Patients: A Handbook for Ward Sisters*, HMSO, London.

Block, D. (1977) Criteria, standards, norms. *Journal of Nursing Administration*, **7**(7), 19–30.

Bowman, M.P. (1986) *Nursing Management and Education: A Conceptual Approach to Change*, Croom Helm, London.

Breemhaar, B., Visser, A.P. and Kleijnen, J.G.V.M. (1990) Perceptions and behaviour among elderly hospital patients: description and explanation of age differences in satisfaction, knowledge, emotions and behaviour. *Social Science and Medicine*, **31**(12), 1377–85.

Briggs, A. (Chairman) (1972) *Report of the Committee on Nursing* (Cm. 5115), HMSO, London.

Department of Health Nursing Division (1989) *A Strategy for Nursing* (A report of the Steering Committee), Department of Health, Nursing Division, London.

Department of Health (1991) *The Patients' Charter*, HMSO, London.

Kitson, A, (1990) *Quality Patient Care: An Introduction to the Dynamic Standards Setting System*, RCN, London.

Kraegel, J.M. *et al.* (1972) A system of care based on patient needs. *Nursing Outlook*, **20**(4), 257–64.

Mayeroff, M. (1971) *On Caring*, Harper & Row, New York.

Merrison, A. (Chairman) (1979) *Royal Commission on the National Health Service* (Cm. 7615), HMSO, London.

Moores, B. and Thompson, A.G.H. (1986) What 1537 hospital inpatients think about aspects of their stay in British acute hospitals. *Journal of Advnced Nursing*, **11**, 87–102.

National Health Service and Community Care Act 1990, HMSO, London.

NHS Management Executive (1992) *One Year On: The Nurse Executive Director Post* (Report on the role and function of the nurse executive director post in first wave NHS trusts), Department of Health, London.

Orem, D.E. (1985) *Nursing, Concepts of Practice*, 3rd edn, McGraw-Hill, New York.

Powell, M. (Chairman) (1966) *The Post-certificate Training and Education of Nurses*, HMSO, London.

Roper, N. *et al.* (1985) *Principles of Nursing*, 3rd edn, Churchill Livingstone, Edinburgh.

Royal College of Nursing of the United Kingdom (1980) *Standards of Nursing Care* (A discussion document), RCN, London.

Royal College of Nursing of the United Kingdom (1981) *Towards Standards* (A discussion document), The second report of the RCN working committee on standards of nursing care, (England and Wales), RCN, London.

Seccombe, I. and Ball, J. (1992) *Motivation, Morale and Mobility: A Profile of Qualified Nurses in the 1990s* (IMS Report No. 233), RCN, London.

United Kingdom Central Council for Nursing, Midwifery and Health Visiting (1992a)

Code of Professional Conduct for the Nurse, Midwife and Health Visitor, UKCC, London.

United Kingdom Central Council for Nursing, Midwifery and Health Visiting (1992b) *The Scope of Professional Practice*, UKCC, London.

World Health Organization (1966) *WHO Expert Committee on Nursing* (fifth report), WHO, Geneva.

Wright-Warren, P. (Chairman) (1986) '*Mix and Match*': *A Review of Skills Mix*, DHSS, London.

Chapter 8

Anderson, E.R. (1973) *The Role of the Nurse* (Royal College of Nursing research project), series 2, No. 1, RCN, London.

Audit Commission (1991) *The Virtue of Patients: Making Best Use of Ward Nursing Resources* (Audit Commission National Health Service Report No. 4), HMSO, London.

Benne, K.D. and Bennis, W. (1959) Role confusion and conflict in nursing: the role of the professional nurse. *American Journal of Nursing*, **LIX**(2), 196–8; (3), 380–3.

Bowman, M.P. (1986) *Nursing Management and Education: A Conceptual Approach to Change*, Croom Helm, Kent.

Briggs, A. (Chairman) (1972) *Report of the Committee on Nursing* (Cm. 5115), HMSO, London.

British Medical Association (1992) *Stress and the Medical Profession*, BMA, London.

Bunge, C.A. (1989) Stress in the library workplace. *Library Trends*, **38**(1), 92–102.

Cattell, R.B. and Ebel, H.W. (1964) *Handbook for the Sixteen Personality Questionnaire*, Institute for Personality and Ability Testing, USA.

Cooper, C.L. and Marshall, J. (eds), (1980) *White Collar and Professional Stress*, John Wiley & Sons, Chichester.

Cooper, C.L. and Roden, J. (1985) Mental health and satisfaction among tax officers. *Social Science and Medicine*, **21**(7), 747–51.

Cooper, C.L., Rout, U. and Faragher, B. (1989) Mental health, job satisfaction, and job stress among general practitioners. *British Medical Journal*, **298**, 366–70.

Cooper, C.L. and Watts, J. (1987) Job satisfaction, mental health and job stressors among general dental practice in the UK. *General Dental Practice*, **24**, 77–81.

Currie, D. (1992) *Stress in the Health Service (South-Central England)*, Southampton Institute of Higher Education, Southampton.

English National Board for Nursing, Midwifery and Health Visiting (1992) Framework for continuing professional education and higher award. *ENB News*, **Spring/Summer/Autumn**.

Eysenck, H.J. (1963) *The Eysenck Personality Inventory*, Educational and Industrial Testing Service, University of London Press, London.

Finnegan, M.J. *et al.* (1984) The sick building syndrome: prevalence studies. *British Medical Journal*, **289**, 1573–5.

Gray-Toft, P. and Anderson, J.G. (1981) Stress among hospital nursing staff: its causes and effects. *Social Sciences and Medicine*, **15A**(5), 639–47.

Guide Dogs for the Blind Association (1993) *GDBA Technical Review*, March 1993, Hillfields, Burghfield Common, Reading, Berkshire.

Hardy, M.E. and Conway, M.E. (1978) *Role Theory: Perspectives for Health Professionals*, Appleton-Century Croft, New York.

Hingley, P. *et al.* (1984) *Stress in Nurse Managers* (Project paper number 60), King Edward Hospitals Fund, London.

Katz, D. and Kahn, R.L. (1978) *The Social Psychology of Organizations*, 2nd edn, John Wiley and Sons, New York.

Khan, H. and Cooper, C.L. (1990) Mental health, job satisfaction, alcohol intake and occupational stress among dealers in financial markets. *Stress Medicine*, **6**, 285–98.

Marmot, M.G. *et al.* (1991) Health inequalities among British civil servants: The Whitehall 11 Study, *Lancet*, **337**, 1387–93.

Marshall, J. (1980) Stress among nurses, in *White Collar and Professional Stress*, (eds C.L. Cooper and J. Marshall), Wiley, Chichester.

MIND (1992) *The MIND Survey: Stress at Work*, National Association for Mental Health, London.

Ostler, J. and Oon, J.T. (1989) The sources of stress and satisfaction in one academic library. *College and Research Library News*, **7**, 587–9.

Owen, G. (1989) *National Association for Staff Support (NASS)*, Surrey, England.

Revans, R.W. (1964) *Standards for Morale: Cause and Effect in Hospitals*, Oxford University Press, Oxford.

Royal College of Nursing of the United Kingdom (1993) *Counselling Help and Advice Together (CHAT)*, RCN, London.

Seccombe, I. and Ball, J. (1992) *Motivation, Morale and Mobility: A Profile of Qualified Nurses in the 1990's* (IMS Report No. 233), RCN, London.

Sykes, J.M. (1988) *Sick Building Syndrome: A Review*, Health and Safety Executive, Merseyside.

The Times (1857) Hospital nurses. *The Times*, London, April 15, p. 6.

Travers, C.J. and Cooper, C.L. (1991) Stress and status in teaching: an investigation of potential gender-related relationships. *Women in Management: Review and Abstracts*, **6**(4), 16–23.

Travers, C.J. and Cooper, C.L. (1992) *Mental Health, Job Satisfaction and Occupational Stress among UK Teachers*, Research sponsored by the National Association of Schoolmasters and Union of Women Teachers.

United Kingdom Central Council for Nursing, Midwifery and Health Visiting (1986) *Project 2000* (report), UKCC, London.

United Kingdom Central Council for Nursing, Midwifery and Health Visiting (1987) *Project 2000: Report on the Costs, Benefits and Manpower Implications of Project 2000* (Price Waterhouse), UKCC, London.

United Kingdom Central Council for Nursing, Midwifery and Health Visiting (1992) *Code of Professional Conduct*, UKCC, London.

Wieland, G.F. (ed) (1981) *Improving Health Care Management: Organization Development and Organization Change*, Health Administration Press, Ann Arbor, Michigan.

World Health Organization Regional Office for Europe (1982) *Indoor Air Pollutants: Exposure and Health Effects* (Report on a WHO meeting, Norlingen), WHO, pp. 8–11.

Chapter 9

Argaris, C. (1985) *Strategy, Change and Defensive Routines*, Pitman, Marsh Field.

Audit Commission (1991) *The Virtue of Patients: Making Best Use of Ward Nursing Resources*, HMSO, London.

Audit Commission (1992) *Making time for Patients: A Handbook for Ward Sisters*, HMSO, London.

Bennis, W.G. (1966) *Changing Organizations*, McGraw-Hill, New York.

Bowman, M.P. (1990) An exploration of the role of the nurse in acute medical and surgical and longstay (geriatric) wards, unpublished PhD thesis submitted to the University of Newcastle upon Tyne, Newcastle upon Tyne.

Briggs, A.D. (Chairman) (1972) *Report on the Committee on Nursing* (Cm. 5115), HMSO, London.

Bruner, J. (1977) *The Process of Education*, Harvard University Press, USA.

Butler, J. (1992) *Patients, Policies and Politics: Before and after Working for Patients*, Open University Press, Buckingham, England.

Chronically Sick and Disabled Persons Act 1970 (Chapter 44), HMSO, London.

Chronically Sick and Disabled Persons (Amendment) Act 1976 (Chapter 49), HMSO, London.

Cooper, C.L. (1981) *Psychology and Management*, Macmillan, London.

Department of Health (1989) *Caring for People: Community Care in the Next Decade and Beyond* (Cm. 849), HMSO, London.

Department of Health (1989) *Working for Patients* (White Paper) (Cm. 555), HMSO, London.

Department of Health (1989) *Self-governing Hospitals: An Initial Guide*, HMSO, London.

Department of Health (1991) *Patient's Charter*, HMSO, London.

Department of Health (1992) *One Year On: The Nurse Executive Director*, Central Office of Information, London.

Department of Health and Social Security (1983) *Nurse Manpower. Planning: Approaches and Techniques*, HMSO, London.

Department of Health, Nursing Division (1989) *A Strategy for Nursing* (a report of the Steering Committee), Department of Health, London.

Department of Health, Scottish Home and Health Department, Welsh Office, Department of Health and Social Services Northern Ireland (1989) *Review of the UKCC and the Four National Boards for Nursing, Midwifery and Health Visiting* (Peat, Marwick, McLintock Report), DSS, London.

Disabled Persons (Services, Consultation and Representation) Act 1986 (Chapter 33), HMSO, London.

Dixon, B. (1992) Professional framework for higher award. *ENB News*, **4** (Spring).

Drucker, P.F. (1980) *Managing in Turbulent Times*, Pan Books, London.

English National Board for Nursing, Midwifery and Health Visiting (1992a) *ENB News*, **5** (Summer).

English National Board for Nursing, Midwifery and Health Visiting (1992b) *ENB News*, **5** (Autumn).

English National Board for Nursing, Midwifery and Health Visiting (1992c) *ENB News*, **5** (Winter).

English National Board for Nursing, Midwifery and Health Visiting (1993a) *Total

Students in Training as at 31 March 1993: Regional Summaries: Pre-registration Nursing, ENB, London.

English National Board for Nursing, Midwifery and Health Visiting (1993b) *The Provision of Learning Experiences in the Community for Project 2000 Students (Research Highlights Two)*, ENB, London.

European Economic Community (1977) Nursing directives 77/452/EEC, 77/453/EEC, 77/454/EEC. *Official Journal of the European Communities*, **July**, L176, 11–12.

European Economic Community (1989) Nursing directives 89/594/EEC. *Official Journal of the European Communities*, **November**, L341, 19.

Foster, H (1992) *ENB News*, **4** (Spring).

Fulmer, R.M. (1988) *The New Management*, 4th edn, Macmillan, New York.

Griffiths, R. (Chairman) (1983) *National Health Service Inquiry*, DHSS, London.

Guide Dogs for the Blind Association (1993) Teaching the teachers. *Forward Magazine*, **March**, Reading, Berkshire.

Hackett, D.W. (1993) Editorial. *Management Today*, **June**, 3.

Hardy, M.E. and Conway, M.E. (1978) *Role Theory: Perspectives for Health Professionals*, Appleton-Century Croft, New York.

Hunt, G. (1992) Project 2000: ethics, ambivalence and ideology, in *Project 2000: The Teachers Speak*, (eds O. Slevin and M. Buckenham), Campion Press, Edinburgh.

Hunt, G. (1993) Misguided attempts at tackling poor quality care. *Nursing Standard*, **7**(34), 12–18.

Jowett, S. *et al.* (1991) *The NFER Project 2000 Research: (Paper No. 2) An Introduction and Some Interim Issues*, National Foundation for Educational Research, Berkshire.

Jowett, S. *et al.* (1992) *Implementing Project 2000: An Interim Report*, National Foundation for Educational Research, Berkshire.

Jowett, S. *et al.* (1994) *Challenges and Change in Nurse Education – A Study of the Implementation of Project 2000*, National Foundation for Educational Research, Berkshire.

Judge, H. (Chairman) (1985) *The Education of Nurses: A New Dispensation* (Commission on Nursing Education), RCN, London.

Kingman, S. (1993) The Freeman Hospital: disillusionment sets in. *British Medical Journal*, **306**(6890), 1464–7.

Kramer, M.F. (1974) *Reality Shock: Why Nurses Leave Nursing*, C.V. Mosby, Saint Louis.

Leonard, A. and Jowett, S. (1990) *Project 2000: Charting the Course* (a study of the 6 ENB pilot schemes in pre-registration nurse education), National Foundation for Educational Research, Berkshire.

Loveridge, R. and Pitt, M. (eds) (1990) *The Strategic Management of Technological Innovation*, Wiley and Sons, Chichester.

Mangham, I.L. (1988) *Effecting Organizational Change*, Blackwell, Oxford.

Mauksch, I. and Miller, M.H. (1981) *Implementing Change in Nursing*, C.V. Mosby, Saint Louis.

Merrison, A. (Chairman) (1979) *Royal Commission on the National Health Service* (Cm. 7615), HMSO, London.

Moores, B. and Thompson, A.G.H. (1986) What 1357 hospital in-patients think about aspects of their stay in British acute hospitals. *Journal of Advance Nursing*, **11**(i), 87–102.

National Audit Office (1985) *National Health Service: Control of Nursing Manpower*, HMSO, London.

National Health Service and Community Care Act 1990 (Chapter 19), HMSO, London.

Nurses, Midwives and Health Visitors Act 1979 (Chapter 36), HMSO, London.

Nurses, Midwives and Health Visitors Rules Approval Order (1983), No. 873, HMSO, London.

Office of Population Censuses and Surveys (1989) *Survey on Disability*, OPCS, London.

O'Reilly, B. (1993) How executives learn now. *Fortune International*, **127**(7).

Pembrey, S. (1980) *The Ward Sister – Key to Nursing* (RCN research report), RCN, London.

Revans, R.W. (1983) *ABC of Action Learning*, Chartwell-Bratt, Kent.

Rowbottom, R. and Billis, D. (1987) *Organisational Design*, Gower, Hants.

Royal College of Nursing of the United Kingdom (1988) *Boundaries of Nursing: A Policy Statement*, RCN, London.

Royal College of Nursing of the United Kingdom (1990) *Resourcing Project 2000 – the Role of Libraries*, RCN, London.

Royal National Institute for the Blind (1991) *Needs Survey (Blind and Partially Sighted Adults in Britain* (Vol. 1), HMSO, London.

Salmon, B. (Chairman) (1966) *Committee on Senior Nursing Staff Structure*, Ministry of Health Scottish Home and Health Department, London.

Seccombe, I. and Buchan, J. *Absent Nurses: The Costs and Consequences* (IMS report 250), RCN, London.

Twiss, B. (1992) *Managing Technological Innovation*, 4th edn, Pitman, London.

United Kingdom Central Council for Nursing, Midwifery and Health Visiting (1986) *Project 2000: A New Preparation for Practice*, UKCC, London.

United Kingdom Central Council for Nursing, Midwifery and Health Visiting (1987) *Project 2000: Report on the Costs, Benefits and Manpower Implications of Project 2000* (Price Waterhouse), UKCC, London.

United Kingdom Central Council for Nursing, Midwifery and Health Visiting (1992) *Code of Professional Conduct*, UKCC, London.

United Kingdom Central Council for Nursing, Midwifery and Health Visiting (1992) *The Scope of Professional Practice*, UKCC, London.

Warwick, D. (1987) *The Modular Curriculum*, Blackwell, Oxford.

Warwick, D. (1988) *Teaching and Learning through Modules*, Blackwell, Oxford.

Index

Page numbers appearing in **bold** refer to figures and page numbers appearing in *italic* refer to tables.